Health Humanities

Health Humanities

Paul Crawford
Professor of Health Humanities, University of Nottingham, UK

Brian Brown
Professor of Health Communication, De Montfort University, UK

Charley Baker
Lecturer in Mental Health, University of Nottingham, UK

Victoria Tischler
Senior Lecturer in Psychology, University of the Arts, London, London College of Fashion, UK

and

Brian Abrams
Associate Professor, Montclair State University, USA

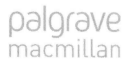
palgrave
macmillan

First published 2015 by
PALGRAVE MACMILLAN

Palgrave Macmillan in the UK is an imprint of Macmillan Publishers Limited, registered in England, company number 785998, of Houndmills, Basingstoke, Hampshire RG21 6XS.

Palgrave Macmillan in the US is a division of St Martin's Press LLC, 175 Fifth Avenue, New York, NY 10010.

Palgrave Macmillan is the global academic imprint of the above companies and has companies and representatives throughout the world.

Palgrave® and Macmillan® are registered trademarks in the United States, the United Kingdom, Europe and other countries.

ISBN 978-1-137-28260-6   ISBN 978-1-137-28261-3 (eBook)
DOI 10.1057/9781137282613

A catalogue record for this book is available from the British Library.

Library of Congress Cataloging-in-Publication Data
Crawford, Paul, 1963– , author.
Health humanities / Paul Crawford, Brian Brown, Charley Baker, Victoria Tischler, Brian Abrams.
p. ; cm.
Includes bibliographical references.
ISBN 978-1-137-28260-6

I. Brown, Brian, 1962– , author. II. Baker, Charley, 1981– , author.
III. Tischler, Victoria, 1968– , author. IV. Abrams, Brian, author. V. Title.
[DNLM: 1. Philosophy, Medical. 2. Health Personnel—education.
3. Humanities. W 61]
R723
610.1—dc23

2014038800

Typeset by MPS Limited, Chennai, India.

For Jamie, Ruby and Owen

Contents

List of Figures and Tables

Figures

Table

Acknowledgements

The authors are very grateful to the Arts and Humanities Research Council (AHRC) for providing successive funding for the health humanities. Early on, such funding [AH/G00968611; AH/J00220811] supported the creation of the Madness and Literature Network (MLN) and International Health Humanities Network (IHHN), respectively. The work of MLN was further advanced by The Leverhulme Trust who funded an investigation into post-war British and American representation of madness. More recently, major AHRC/Research Councils UK (RCUK) funding [AH/K00336411] established a national consortium investigating creative practice as mutual recovery as part of the Connected Communities programme. We would like to thank all members of the Creative Practice as Mutual Recovery consortium for helping to develop an increasingly rich understanding of 'mutual recovery', as discussed in Chapter 8. We would also like to thank all members and associates of the Centre for Social Futures at the Institute of Mental Health and Centre for Advanced Studies, The University of Nottingham. Thanks also go to Martin Stott, Neil Robinson and Nick Palmer for stalwart work in bringing policy ears to health humanities. Finally, we would like to thank our many compatriots across the globe – far too many now to mention individually – who have joined the health humanities club and lead and inspire new and exciting developments!

About the Authors

Paul Crawford is the world's first Professor of Health Humanities and has been the leading figure in developing the field of health humanities worldwide. He is Principal Investigator for the AHRC-funded International Health Humanities Network (IHHN), Madness and Literature Network (MLN) and the Creative Practice as Mutual Recovery programme and leads the International Health Humanities Conference series, bringing substantial teams of interdisciplinary scholars together. He directs both Nottingham Health Humanities and Centre for Social Futures at the Institute of Mental Health/ School of Health Sciences, The University of Nottingham, UK. In 2013 he was made a Fellow of the prestigious Academy of Social Sciences for his work in advancing applied linguistics in healthcare and is also a Fellow of the Royal Society of Arts.

Brian Brown is Professor of Health Communication at De Montfort University, UK. The core of his work has focused on the interpretation of human experience across a variety of different disciplines including healthcare, philosophy, education and spirituality studies, exploring how this may be understood with a view to improving practice and with regard to theoretical development in the social sciences. Particularly, this concerns notions of governmentality and habitus from Foucauldian and Bourdieusian sociology and how the analysis of everyday experience can afford novel theoretical developments.

Charley Baker is Lecturer in Mental Health at the School of Health Sciences at The University of Nottingham where she teaches mental health nursing students at BSc level and on the Graduate Entry Nursing programme. She is lead author of the co-authored monograph *Madness in Post-1945 British and American Fiction* (Palgrave, 2010) and co-founded the IHHN and MLN. She has a BA and MA in literature and is working on her PhD on psychosis and postmodernism at Royal Holloway, University of London. She is also Associate Editor of *Journal of Psychiatric and Mental Health Nursing* and serves on the editorial board of *Journal of Medical Humanities*.

Victoria Tischler is Senior Lecturer in Psychology at the University of the Arts, London, London College of Fashion. Her research interests concern the use of creative approaches in mental health care. She teaches psychology applied to fashion. She is also a curator and has developed exhibitions focused on the medico-historical significance of art created in asylums.

Brian Abrams is Associate Professor of Music and Coordinator of Music Therapy at Montclair State University, New Jersey, USA. He is an Analytical Music Therapist and Fellow of the Association for Music and Imagery. He has been a music therapist since 1995, with experience across a wide range of clinical contexts. His research has included topics such as music therapy in cancer care, music psychotherapy, humanistic music therapy, and the interdisciplinary area of health humanities. He has also contributed to the establishment of several medical music therapy programmes and served on editorial boards of numerous journals and as President of the American Music Therapy Association (AMTA).

1
Health Humanities

There is a growing need for a new kind of debate at the intersection of the humanities and healthcare, health and well-being. In the recent past the field of medical humanities has grown rapidly, but it is timely and appropriate to address the increasing and broadening demand from other professions to become involved, to accommodate new sectors of the healthcare workforce and the public, and to extend 'appliedness' in relation to how arts and humanities knowledge and practices can inform and transform healthcare, health and well-being. There are important cohorts of personnel in healthcare, a whole army of ancillary workers, as well as informal carers and patients themselves who have been largely left out of the medical humanities so far. Moreover, as different disciplines come to value the contribution made by the arts and humanities and new opportunities emerge in health for the development and inclusion of new approaches here, it is important that this expansion and debate is given voice and new fora are created for these new developments.

The so-called medical humanities were the first on the scene, and have developed strongly in the Anglophone world. But now the field of health humanities, subsuming arts within the term 'humanities', is fast developing a more inclusive and international capture of material as other disciplines and different nations develop their own distinctive practice and theory. Its expansion is marked by health humanities-focused research funding calls, dedicated centres and networks, and changes to existing medical humanities centres to align with health humanities, either in their more inclusive names or programmes of work. For example, we hear increased reference to

1

'medical and health humanities' or even 'medical health humanities'. But not everyone aligns with medical visions of healthcare or giving it this kind of primacy or privilege in new terminological marriages. Furthermore, there are multiple and often complementary contributions to health and well-being which fall outside medicine per se. In other words, medicalised humanities are not the only show in town. With increased consideration of the emergence of health humanities in the UK, US and Canada and resultant new inflections of medical humanities as 'critical medical humanities', as in Bates et al. (2014), all this merits a new publication aiming to give a flavour of the diverse range of healthcare activities and the newly discovered relationships between these and the humanities themselves. Indeed, the rise of the more inclusive health humanities marks an evolution of medical humanities.

Health humanities is marked by an ambition for the following:

- new combinations of pedagogic approaches informed by the arts and humanities in education of all professional personnel involved in healthcare, health and well-being
- advancing the health and well-being benefits of involvement in arts and humanities to informal or unpaid carers/caretakers and the self-caring public
- valuing and sustaining existing therapeutic applications of arts and humanities to the benefit of any nation's health and social well-being
- democratising therapeutic interventions whenever possible and feasible beyond specialist professionals
- championing increased sharing of the arts and humanities capacities and resources of the professional health workforce, informal carers and patients themselves in enhancing healthcare environments.

It is tempting to see the growth of interest from scholars and practitioners in the humanities in healthcare as being spearheaded by the medical humanities, an area which has recently been described as having gained the status of a 'mature discipline' (Ahlzen, 2007). Certainly, this area has been influential and has recently gained ground as an alternative to the traditional, exclusively scientific curriculum pursued in the English-speaking world and many postcolonial nations. Changes in medical education were prompted by re-evaluations from educators and professional bodies on both sides of the Atlantic through the 1990s (Christakis, 1995; Enarson and Burg, 1992; General Medical Council, 1993; Schwarz and Wojtczak, 2002). This has involved a great deal of questioning of medical school curricula and a reappraisal of the kinds of qualities that educators are attempting to foster in tomorrow's health professionals. This in turn has led to opportunities for the development of curricula for healthcare professions to include the humanities. Classically, in the case of medicine, this has involved ethics or 'moral attitude' (Olthuis and Dekkers, 2003) or confronting students with some of the enigmas or conundrums of the discipline to make them aware of philosophical issues (Brawer, 2006). More recently this has broadened to include literature (Dysart-Gale, 2008), expanding clinical empathy (Garden, 2009), dealing with the more exasperating experiences of clinical life (Gordon, 2008), as well as developing community education and a commitment to interdisciplinarity (Donohoe and Danielson, 2004). In addition we have seen a focus on both medicine and the humanities as interpretive enterprises (Gillis, 2008), or recognition of healthcare practice as a kind of performance, analogous to being a musician (Woolliscroft and Phillips, 2003). The intention is that medicine should reconfigure its boundaries to become interdisciplinary and at the same time become disciplined through the humanities on the premise that 'arts and humanities approaches can foster significant interpretive enquiry into illness, disability, suffering, and care' (Bolton, 2008, p. 131). The notion of 'humanities' itself suggests a shared understanding of what it means to be 'humane', either as a person or as interpersonal practice. Some of the purported benefits of teaching medical humanities include the promotion of patient-centred care, combatting professional burnout and 'equipping doctors to meet moral challenges not "covered" by biomedicine' (Gordon, 2005; Petersen et al., 2008, p. 2). Yet this diversity of claimed benefits is often as confusing as it is comprehensive. Thus, there are those who point to the lack of consensus as to what exactly constitutes medical humanities and what the discipline is for (Petersen et al., 2008).

Despite this apparent hegemony of medicine, as we shall see in the present volume, medicine does not have exclusive claim upon the action. We intend to outline how a variety of other disciplines have sought to incorporate the arts and humanities, or have attempted to relate the arts and humanities to practitioner education, practice with clients, professional development and the wider development of the discipline. The hitherto more narrowly defined medical humanities therefore do not necessarily have a monopoly over the work undertaken. In particular, the vast body of practical work undertaken globally in the expressive therapies demands and deserves admission to the health humanities. Here, practitioners and researchers are often actively seeking places where they can develop ideas and place them on a more theoretically mature footing, as well as providing a means of bringing this work more fully to the attention of scholars in the medical humanities, those in practice, and those who teach the health professionals of the future.

In this chapter therefore we propose to provide a brief tour through some of the developments in the humanities and arts throughout healthcare. Whilst not an exhaustive summary, we should be able to provide the reader with some indications of how diverse disciplines have attempted to incorporate the humanities, and how humanities scholars have built the healthcare disciplines into their purview.

One of the key concerns linking the healthcare disciplines and the humanities is the notion of meaning. In a variety of healthcare settings, meaning plays a central role in the effort to understand the individual's life-world (Kvale, 1996), and as Stetler (2010) adds, their personal and social realities, patterns of action and behaviour. A consideration of meaning is central to both the humanities and healthcare because people ascribe specific values and purpose to their experiences, conduct and relationships. Matters are made meaningful when people understand and make sense of their actions, feelings and thoughts. Often this occurs through people creating narratives about themselves and events in their world. This understanding involves a continuous interpretative process which is informed by the individual's prior knowledge, experiences, emotions, beliefs and attitudes. As Stetler (2010) notes, this process forms the individual's current sense of reality.

The distinctive contribution of the humanities, as disciplines that have often been at the forefront of interpreting human experience, is perhaps most pronounced where the notion of meaning is concerned. This is perhaps easiest to appreciate if we remind ourselves of the distinction between 'meaning' and 'information'. Human beings seldom function in a way which is directly like computers as they process information or data. This difference was emphasised by Jerome Bruner (1990), an influential advocate of a culture- and action-orientation in the study of thinking and experience. According to Bruner, rather than being best conceived of as 'data processing devices', it is more appropriate to consider human beings as continually seeking meaning, interpreting their environment, other individuals and themselves in a process of dynamic interaction with the world around them. As Stetler (2010) says, meaning therefore can be understood as a dynamic, situational and dialogical concept.

This grounding of meaning in interaction and dialogue places it firmly in the territory of the humanities. As Gendlin puts it, 'meaning is formed in the interaction of experiencing and is something that functions as a symbol' (Gendlin, 1997, p. 8). This process of symbolisation is often undertaken through the use of the spoken word, but can also be expressed by other means, such as movement, art, sculpture, performance, thinking or writing. Equally, the way that all these activities are actualised or realised through the body places the healthcare disciplines – with their preoccupation with bodily matters – clearly in the scope of meaning-making. For Merleau-Ponty (1962) it is through the lived body that we anchor ourselves to the world. Elaine Scarry (1985) goes further. For her the body's capacity to suffer is fundamental to the construction of culture and society. Our pain, she suggests, is at once the most irreducible of subjective experiences and the most incommunicable. For example, pain is rarely rendered in detail in most novels, yet haunts the warp and weft of human cultures.

Meaning, then, is often embodied, but it is also contextualised. In Bruner's (1990) view, meaning always emerges as something that is formed in situated action. In this sense, meaning is a reflective response to being involved and in action; in other words meaning is about doing things. As Giddens (1991, p. 284) says, in the human disciplines we are confronted with 'phenomena which are already constituted as meaningful. The condition of "entry" to this field is getting to know what actors already know, and have to know, to "go on" in the daily activities of social life'. Bruner saw meaning-making as foundational to the creation of human cultures, and the proper conduct of the human disciplines as being to elicit insights about how the participants who are involved in culture make sense of it.

The notion of meaning integrates past, present and future. Meaning is created on the basis of traces of earlier experience which the individual deploys to entrain and interrogate the current situation, and meaning also emerges through the incorporation of a possible or expected future into the current action. As part of this meaning-making process, the meanings derived from the sensory data of experience are shaped through social negotiation and narratives (Polkinghorne, 1988) that describe and are grounded in the social actor's thoughts, feelings and reflections on their life practice. In an important sense this form of meaning-making is cultural or collective and results from the social, co-creative interaction between humans as social beings. One important role of the arts and humanities in healthcare is to dramatically expand the scope of the social negotiations and verbal or visual narratives available as we make sense of health and illness. It is through the arts and humanities that we have access to the meanings, narratives, adjudications and interventions of a multitude of other people across the broad sweep of history and different cultures. The arts and humanities rescue us from the sometimes stultifying localism or myopia of a particular discipline or social situation. In healthcare, stories, novels and poetry can illustrate a huge range of social and health problems from the perspective of the writer (Calman, 2005). Similarly, music, art, drama and a multitude of many other kinds of creative expression and craft can narrate health and illness experience and viewpoints. Within the medical humanities, as Charon (2006a, p. 191) points out, doctors have for a long time been turning to literary texts and ways of thinking that help us to enter the subjective worlds of patients, see others' experience from their own perspectives, appreciate the metaphorical as well as the straightforward communicative power of words, and be moved by what we hear.

This scope for stories to enhance and liberate our experience whether we are patients, carers or health professionals is underscored by Sarbin (1997, p. 67), in his article 'The poetics of identity', where he argues that 'imaginings influence the construction of identity ... that imaginings stimulated by stories read or stories heard can provide the plot structures for one's own self-narratives'. As Diekman et al. go on to argue, 'fiction's narrative form and its ability to transport the reader into a vivid and involving fictional world are powerful persuasive tools in and of themselves' (Diekman et al., 2000, p. 180).

Indeed, earlier work suggests that the more people feel 'transported' by their reading, the more likely they are to be persuaded by it (Green and Brock, 1996). Even when stories are fictional, they play a vital role in enabling readers to form beliefs and expectations around their reading (Diekman et al., 2000), implying that fiction may be an influential mechanism for changing health practice and health behaviour. Of course, we need to retain awareness that not all storytelling is read or heard – for example, storytelling, digital or otherwise, can be achieved in individual, successive or moving images.

Therefore, the notion of meaning is central to the project of the health humanities. The human context of suffering and healing is uniquely susceptible to illumination by literature and the arts, irrespective of the particular health specialisms involved. Indeed, it is the search for meaning and integration in patients' experiences which brings together often disparate points of view on a condition. As Stetler (2010) goes on to argue, meaning has both a social and a narrative dimension. Through the incorporation of multiple stories, meaning can develop a dynamic quality which is not exclusively based on the participant's experiences, but evolves in a process of co-creation, where the individual responds to those around him or her as well as the stories they encounter. In an important sense then, meaning in healthcare is a joint construction, created, as Swanson (1992) maintains, through people doing things together. In this sense, the concept of meaning is the result of the integration of the experiential, pre-reflective dimension with the discursive, narrative dimension.

The social world, including the social world of healthcare, is always meaningfully pre-interpreted and meaning is constitutive of social phenomena (Schutz, 1962). For a number of key thinkers concerned with the human condition, from Max Weber to Alfred Schutz, it is meaning that distinguishes between a mere probabilistic relationship between cause and effect and a genuinely explanatory understanding (Eberele, 2010). In the healthcare disciplines this is no less so than in the social sciences. In the contemporary idiom, meaning is one of the major 'trending topics' in present-day medical research, with an increase in attention to existential, spiritual and religious issues in relation to illness (La Cour and Hvidt, 2010).

Meaning is intimately bound up with what we do, how we use words and images or other media, deploy techniques and act on the world around us. As Wittgenstein famously claimed, 'the meaning is the use' and that understanding the meaning of something involves being able to continue our course of action – 'now I know how to go on' (Wittgenstein, 1953). Meaning, like healthcare itself, is therefore often about doing things together. And in doing things we are often engaged, literally and metaphorically, in using tools. From equipment itself to particular ways of thinking and talking, the use of tools and technologies is ubiquitous. There is a reciprocal relationship between the tools humans invent and the social, representational and relational systems that emerge and co-constitute our development. As Vygotsky (1978) argued, the mediating signs and artefacts people use to understand and represent the experiential world form a generative basis for human experience, social life and culture. Within individuals' consciousness, encounters with the uses and meanings of these signs and artefacts give rise to interpersonal, collective mental structures and processes (Toulmin, 1978). In Vygotsky's view, the tools we construct and use to mediate these symbolic activities change the ways humans think. By building tools, people build the material basis for consciousness, transforming the environments and restructuring the functional systems in which they act and learn (Vygotsky, 1978; Wartofsky, 1983). In so doing, they launch developmental trajectories of thought and action that resonate broadly, spanning dimensions of the individual and the collective, the material and the symbolic.

Fundamental to the idea of health humanities is the assumption that it is through the arts and humanities then that we can fully grasp the meaning of events and experiences in healthcare. Moreover, it is through the arts and humanities that we can also come to an understanding of the effects that technologies, tools, techniques and health-related ways of thinking have upon us. Echoing Clemenceau's comments about war, one might even say that health is too important to be left to the doctors. The arts and humanities represent a wealth of experience in musing upon the human condition and in thinking critically about texts and images, be they literary, scientific or part of the burgeoning genres of health education advice or self-help – thinking about how human beings are conceptualised and constructed, how we are persuaded of courses of action, how the science of health fits into a historical or political context. Thinking about the conceptualisations, presuppositions and epistemological commitments of healthcare is not to do away with them, but rather, as Judith Butler (1993, p. 30) puts it, to free them from their 'metaphysical lodgings in order to understand what political interests were secured in and by that metaphysical placing'. In other words, we can be empowered to question the apparent certainty and epistemological privilege of healthcare knowledge. As Butler (1993, p. 30) goes on to say, 'to problematize the matter of bodies may entail an initial loss of epistemological certainty, but a loss of certainty is not the same as political nihilism ... the unsettling of matter can be understood as initiating new possibilities, new ways for bodies to matter'.

Bodies 'matter', in Butler's sense, across the whole range of healthcare disciplines, and in a variety of areas of practice we can see people applying ideas, techniques and other insights to make sense of what is happening. The arts and humanities have long held a place in nurse education (Dellasega et al., 2007) and a good many researchers and educators in the discipline have deemed it appropriate to include the arts and humanities to inculcate an appreciation of the fullness and complexity of human experience. Moreover, in a reflective fashion, they have been applied to make sense of what nursing is all about. A widely reproduced quotation attributed to Florence Nightingale established the affinity between the arts and nursing:

> Nursing is an art: and if it is to be made an art, it requires an exclusive devotion as hard a preparation, as any painter's or sculptor's work; for what is the having to do with dead canvas or dead marble, compared with having to do with the living body, the temple of God's spirit? It is one of the Fine Arts: I had almost said, the finest of Fine Arts ... there is no such thing as amateur art and there is no such thing as amateur nursing. (McDonald, 2004, pp. 291–292)

There is growing commitment to having a nursing curriculum that involves a full appreciation of the complexity of the human condition (Davis, 2003). Hence, argue Ferrell et al. (2010, p. 941), because nursing is an intrinsically artistic endeavour, as well as a scientific practice, the education of nurses in formal academic programmes and through continuing education for those in practice can be enhanced through inclusion of arts and humanities. Ferrell et al. contend that the humanities and arts are vital to remind nurses that illness is 'a profound human experience' (p. 942) and express the hope that by incorporating the arts into education, practice and professional development, nurses can be moved to a new understanding which engages emotions and self-reflection, enables them to hear and appreciate stories and gain insight into thoughts and experiences that are often repressed. Also in nursing, it is possible to illuminate some of the practices and policies in the present day through analysis of the history of the discipline. For example, Reeves et al. (2010) show how the organisation and regulation of disciplines such as nursing can be traced to the development of 16th-century craft guilds. This has its legacy in the present day where territorial knowledge claims, discipline-specific hierarchies and difficulties in collaborative working can be traced back to the guild-like structure of the different professions in healthcare.

The use of arts and humanities in learning for nurses has also been encouraged by the use of inquiry based learning or problem based learning and the desire to encourage nurses to engage in reflection about their practice where poetry and novels can aid this task, as can reflection about the teaching process itself (McKie et al., 2008, p. 163). There are pleas for the rubric of nursing to extend beyond evidence based practice to include information literacy, the humanities, ethics and the social sciences (Jutel, 2008). Especially in mental health, the arts have been employed as diversional and therapeutic interventions and activities – it is suggested that 'art offers a showing of human experience in unique ways' (Biley and Galvin, 2007, p. 806), and in this way it can facilitate shared understanding of people's experiences.

At the same time as these educational initiatives and pleas for the inclusion of the arts and humanities are going on, there are critical voices raised. For example, Wallace (2008) describes how an appreciation of Henrik Ibsen's *Enemy of the People* helps us gain a critical purchase on the processes of governance in healthcare. The arts and humanities then can assist critical reflection on what is happening to us as human beings in relation to the policies and institutions in which we are embedded. Bishop (2008) challenges the assumption that the humanities should merely exist to make medicine perform 'better' in a narrow technical sense, or provide professionals with 'narrative competencies' that they might otherwise miss acquiring. Instead, he charges, humanities can enable us to challenge this narrow instrumental view of human activity at its very roots. Medical humanism might promise intimacy and care but is it, asks Bishop (2008, p. 21), also about control? This potential to develop a philosophically attuned awareness of what is going on in healthcare offers the opportunity to mount informed critiques and stage novel debates about the meaning of health and healthcare which go beyond the customary question of 'what works'.

In other disciplines too, there are signals that the arts and humanities are being relied upon to play a role. In occupational therapy there were some early signs that literary works were being drawn upon to create reflective discussion (Murray et al., 2000). Occupational therapy has a long history of engagement with the creative arts (Thompson and Blair, 1998), with evidence that this is appreciated by patients, particularly if they are able to set their own goals and terms of engagement (Lim et al., 2007). Especially in mental health and particularly in Australasia, there is a continued emphasis on the role of the arts and creativity in occupational therapy (Schmid, 2004). For example, some of Schmid's participants described using creative activities to look with their clients at issues like hope and inner strength, adaptation and making changes, and developing clients' creativity.

At the same time there is growing interest in creative disciplines such as dance and drama in physiotherapy (Christie et al., 2006). As well as specific manipulations and exercises, there is an increasing appreciation of the patient's life story and narrative in making sense of their experience in therapy. For example, Soundy et al. (2010) show how the process of recovery from a sports injury makes use of a variety of narrative patterns, seeing accounts of injuries and the rehabilitative process as being like a quest, a search for restitution or a lapse into chaos or despair. The value of seeing the larger life context is apparent, and this can be enhanced through the use of stories, life narratives and vignettes in student learning.

The arts and creative therapies as disciplines in their own right have made inroads into fields as diverse as cancer care (Carlson and Bultz, 2008; Puig et al., 2006), mental health care (Perry et al., 2008), including forensic contexts (Smeijsters and Gorry, 2006), dementia care (Mitchell et al., 2006) and social care work with children (Lefevre, 2004). There are lively programmes of innovative practice ongoing in the so-called 'expressive therapies' (Malchiodi, 2006) such as dance therapy (Goodill, 2005; Payne, 2004), poetry therapy (Kempler, 2003; Mazza, 2003), art therapy (Edwards, 2004), art in groupwork settings (Argyle and Bolton, 2004; Liebmann, 2004), psychodrama (Fonseca, 2004) and dramatherapy (Weber and Haen, 2005). This list is not exhaustive, but it should suffice to indicate something of the breadth and nature of the work undertaken across a range of disciplines to introduce the arts and humanities into therapies.

Despite this level of activity, there are still some areas which are relatively unexplored. Notwithstanding their role in the caring process, informal carers are scarcely mentioned in this literature. Whilst we can see the better established therapeutic professions represented, from medical doctors to drama therapists, there is little shrift given to the variety of paraprofessionals and support staff whose efforts contribute to the healthcare experience. Those who provide catering and cleaning services in hospitals may interact with patients and augment the hospital stay but their experiences are so far a terra incognita as far as the humanities are concerned. Likewise, paramedics, ambulance staff and members of charitable or voluntary organisations, despite their substantial contributions, are relatively unknown within the existing medical humanities literature. Crucially, patients or service users themselves as agents of change, or as key contributors to their own recovery as self-helpers, are rarely the focus here.

To sum up the situation briefly, then, there is much work afoot in the medical humanities, and other healthcare disciplines are developing related approaches, but there is still much work to do in cross-fertilising these activities so as to maximise the benefit to practitioners and clients. Equally, there are areas where there is as yet relatively little scholarship but where the arts and humanities are poised to make a contribution, such as exploring the experience of carers, reconnoitring the work of clients and practitioners in roles beyond the relatively narrow set which have so far been explored.

We have ventured into this field and termed it the health humanities, subsuming arts within the term 'humanities', because there is a need to enhance discussion among researchers, practitioners and the public and facilitate educational initiatives so as to build awareness of the role of arts and humanities in education, training and practice across the many fields of health and social care. The new project outlined in this book – the health humanities – is underpinned by several aims. We seek to encourage an inclusive approach which reaches the whole range of activities that go to make up healthcare. We would like to encourage scholarship based on novel practical initiatives in the health humanities, in training, treatment and support for carers and clients. We share a commitment to explore those aspects of healthcare which have hitherto not benefitted from the arts and humanities' perspective, such as paramedical and support staff, informal carers and service users themselves. This new development of a more inclusive field of health humanities is underpinned by a commitment to the thoroughgoing development of critique and critical theory so as to enable the questioning of current practice and also the foundational assumptions of healthcare and the health humanities themselves.

Despite vigorous debate and the conflicting assumptions of different disciplines, practices and foci of attention, there is nevertheless a sense of community between contributors to the humanities in healthcare which over time will benefit not only the field itself but the wider academic and practitioner communities. The new field of the health humanities aims to fill this larger niche which the pioneering medical humanities have begun hollowing out. We seek to create unity among a much larger body of work across different healthcare specialisms and intend that the health humanities as a new field will provide a platform for innovative scholarship upon the range of theory and practice which can link human and artistic studies to the implementation of health and welfare. This more inclusive reach across the whole spectrum of arts, humanities and healthcare activity is intended to embrace not only medicine, but nursing, occupational therapy, dentistry, physiotherapy and social work, as well as the disciplines that have traditionally drawn on the arts and humanities such as dance and drama therapies, poetry therapy, bibliotherapy and the authors' previous experience with storytelling in therapy (Crawford et al., 2004).

Another reason why we have termed our chosen field the heath humanities is that the majority of healthcare as it is practised is non-medical. Despite being a popular activity, visits to the doctor, or doctor consultations in the clinic, are relatively fleeting. Other practitioners and professionals and voluntary sector workers may contribute to care. In hospitals and residential settings clients may spend more time with care assistants, catering and cleaning staff, as well as informal and family carers, than they do with doctors.

In other institutions such as schools, prisons and childcare services, roles are changing and a greater degree of responsibility for the mental and physical health of their charges is expected from practitioners. Complementary and alternative healthcare is growing in popularity and there may be hitherto unexplored ways in which the arts and humanities can help place these in theoretical context and inform practice.

We propose to take a broader view of the arts and humanities, including within our scope literary and critical theory, anthropology, linguistics and other social sciences which have a bearing on the issues under discussion. Whereas there are journals such as *Arts and Health* whose manifesto seeks to explore the arts' role in practice, design and education as these apply to healthcare, we will encourage also the development of theory, concepts and new ways of understanding. The inclusion of critical theory within our ambit will be used to encourage critique, whether in terms of methods, theories, institutions or practices. The traditional ambit of the humanities is to study the human condition often using methods that are analytic, critical or speculative. Language study, literary study, history, theology, visual, performing and multimedia arts, as well as area studies, media and cultural studies, and other aspects of the social sciences which contribute to thought in the humanities form a fertile field of inspiration to scholars and practitioners in healthcare. In addition, novel developments have been taking place at the interface between the humanities and the sciences where the term 'post-human' has been applied. Here there is an emphasis on how humanity can be supplemented or transcended by technology and there are ample points of contact between these accounts and the opportunities afforded by healthcare technology to transcend human limitations and frailties.

As well as living with and through technology, it is also possible for the arts and humanities to enable us to lead richer social lives with consequent advantages in terms of health and well-being. Participation in community activities and creative and recreational programmes supports the development of interpersonal relationships, enhances self-esteem, improves general health, and reduces stress and anxiety in adults and children (Forsyth and Jarvis, 2002; Murphy and Carbone, 2008; Street et al., 2007; Vandell et al., 2005). The creative and performing arts can make valuable contributions to the training of future healthcare professionals such as physiotherapists (Becker and Dusing, 2010), public health and therapy (MacDougall and Yoder, 1998) and medical training (Brodzinski, 2010). All these approaches have attempted to include more practical and experiential learning experiences in the curriculum and to demonstrate the viability of alternatives to conventional classroom learning in the creation of the next generation of health and social care professionals.

Performance has also found its way into the research arena as an approach to research and its dissemination. Based on a research project they had undertaken on the experiences of older women in the south-west of England, Carless and Douglas (2010) describe an initiative to incorporate performances embodying their findings into dissemination strategies. The occasion was their attempt to present their research to audiences including physiotherapy and occupational therapy students. The performance included, and was inspired by, experiences collected through the research on older women, such as visiting Cornwall when they were younger, the love of dancing which several informants had described, and the experience of riding a bicycle which one informant had said made her feel like 'an Arthurian knight off to seek adventure'. Far from being frail and resistant to physical activity, the women in question often described themselves enjoying it and valuing the independence it afforded. Students exposed to this performance as part of their degree course had some mixed feelings. As one said:

> At first I wanted to laugh – because it was something I had never seen, but after a while, it carried me away. I got emotional; and I really enjoyed the way these stories were expressed and the music as well. It is a new experience which attracts all kinds of characters. I believe that this way, it is easier to come close to people you are referring to. Of course it is better because you are able to touch your audience's souls. The song about dance really affected me. Actually all the songs affected me but this particularly, because, you see, it gives you the possibility to bring out images, use your imagination. This affected me because it brought in my mind my grandfather, who didn't dance, but he loved going hunting and a few years ago he stopped because he couldn't walk. That was like the end for him. He died and his dream was to go hunting for the last time. (Carless and Douglas, 2010, pp. 376–377)

Many of our concerns in this volume enjoy a wide currency in education for future healthcare practitioners. Embraced under the rubric
of medical humanities, the subject matter is enjoying increased
coverage in medical schools in the UK, US, Canada and Australasia.
In the UK for example, one estimate of the scale of the audience for
the health humanities can be derived from the universities admis-
sions service UCAS, which lists 31 institutions offering degrees in
medicine and 53 offering degrees in nursing. The North American
continent contains nearly 150 medical schools including the US
and Canada, which are typically educating over 100,000 students at
any one time. The American Association of Medical Colleges (2008)
reported over 18,000 new enrollees in programmes in its accredited
members in 2008. Nursing in the US is served by over 1200 accredited programmes at college level. The US nursing workforce boasts
2.9 million Registered Nurse members, nearly 400,000 of whom
have a doctorate or masters degree (US Department of Health and
Human Services, 2008). Whilst the concern with health humanities is not as far developed in nursing as it is in medicine, the large
numbers of students undertaking advanced study in the profession,
which includes material relating to the philosophy of the discipline,
a variety of research methods and elements of history and philosophy of science suggests a large and growing demand for educational
resources. This is especially opportune as the US government seeks
to increase training places and postgraduate education for nurses to
meet the shortage of nursing personnel in the United States today.

Hence, we can get a sense of the scale of the healthcare workforce,
especially in the US, and the likely demand for initiatives that will
allow education in the humanities to be developed for healthcare
personnel. In the US, substantial numbers of academic institutions
are engaged in education and advanced study in medicine and nursing and many institutions make a feature of medical humanities
in their provision. Whilst the situation is changing all the time as
curricula are revised and universities reorganise themselves, the pre-
eminence of the medical humanities is likely to be sustained into the
future and bodes well for the expansion of humanities approaches
into other disciplines.

In most European countries it is expected that students of medicine will know some philosophy. Rather than being ghettoised
into a particular module or specialism, the humanities are more

embedded in the educational culture (Marshall, 2005). A recent issue of the journal *Academic Medicine* reports on humanities programmes in medical education in Europe, highlighting innovations in curriculum design and teaching in a number of European countries. For example the last 10 or so years has seen the development of programmes in Sweden (Ahlzen and Stolt, 2003), Switzerland (Louis-Courvoisier, 2003), Norway (Frich and Fugelli, 2003), and Germany (Kiessling et al., 2003). In the case of Germany, a renewed focus on medical humanities and philosophy came about through student demands and through the shift to problem-based learning. The Norwegian curricular reforms in the 1990s led to the inclusion of music, visual arts, literature and architecture into the medical curriculum and in Croatia, literature and history components are in the curriculum at all the country's medical schools (Fatovic-Ferencic, 2003). These examples should suffice to establish that the medical humanities are thriving in Europe. The historical embeddedness of philosophy and the arts in higher education in Europe means that the ground is prepared for further advances of the health humanities, and expansion into disciplines other than medicine itself is likely to proceed rapidly. It is also set for a telling shift from a largely unitary pedagogic focus to a practical and transformative set of activities and interventions to more directly benefit human health and social experience.

In addition, there is potential interest in the health humanities in many developing parts of the world. To take just a few examples, reports of the demand in this area have emerged from Kathmandu (Adhikari, 2007; Shankar, 2008) and India, as noted by Joshi (2008) who highlights the multitude of faiths and language communities in the country as well as the fact that India is a prime destination for health tourism and pharmaceutical companies seeking to conduct clinical trials. China has recently seen the establishment of a Medical Humanities Institute at Peking University Health Sciences Centre, in October 2008. In Taiwan, a College of Medical Humanities and Social Sciences was established in 2002 at Chungshan Medical University. In South America, Acuna (2000) reports upon two decades of development of the medical humanities in Argentina, where courses include a focus on the arts, literature, history, anthropology and a new discipline, 'medical kalology', or the aesthetics of medicine (Acuna, 2003).

Summary and Conclusions

To summarise this chapter then, the health humanities represent the fusion of a number of humane ways of seeing healthcare, derived from the humanities and the arts. Through much of the last one and a half centuries, a good part of the discipline of medicine has undergone a theoretical and practical shift away from the classical perception of medicine as an art, based on patients' stories of their illnesses, to medicine as a science, based on the doctor's clinical observations and supported by the rapid developments in scientific procedures. The engine house of medicine was no longer in the bedside consultation or in the surgeon's craft, but in the laboratory. To some commentators, this has made medicine seem remote from its human context and has fostered a demand for new ways of looking at the personal and interpersonal processes involved in suffering and healing.

In the health humanities, the arts and humanities are used to provide insight into the human condition, and issues such as suffering, personhood and our responsibility to each other, as well as to offer a historical perspective on healthcare practice itself. Moreover, a key task of this newly emerging field of enquiry is to break down the artificial boundaries between the arts and biomedical science to identify mutually beneficial fields of study. The health humanities, like the medical humanities before them, address the ways in which the humanities disciplines may be involved in exploring more richly-textured ways of understanding healthcare as a practice, and understanding health, illness and care in relation to subjective experience. Moreover, attention to literature and the arts can help develop and nurture skills of observation, analysis, empathy and self-reflection, all of which are involved in humane medical care. The rich insights of the humanities about culture, the body and what it means to be human have direct relevance to clinical practice, as well as facilitating a deeper understanding of how culture interacts with the individual experience of illness and the way healthcare is practised.

The arts and humanities, then, are far too important to be left to medicine alone. Indeed, it is perhaps time for the medical humanities to transform into health humanities or continue to be found wanting by those not limited to a medical vision and keen to see a democratisation of how the arts and humanities can contribute to the health and well-being of the public. Do the health humanities signal the death of medical humanities? It is perhaps too early to pronounce on this but health humanities looks set to become the superordinate term, subsuming medical humanities and other more specific manifestations of congruent work. Already, as a free-form and viral movement, health humanities is beginning to cohere a diverse reach and institutional presence worldwide. This book explores this movement and a range of relevant approaches through the arts and humanities. It does not exclude medical humanities but rather draws it out of its shell to join a more ambitious movement for enrichment and engagement between the arts, humanities and healthcare, health and well-being. Importantly it seeks to see the arts and humanities as a core constituent and enabler of health and well-being by transforming places, processes and people, whether in hospitals, clinics, schools, prisons or community settings. In brief, it begins to outline and illustrate, not least through reference to educational and research case studies, a more inclusive, outward-facing and applied discipline that:

• advances non-professional solutions among informal carers, service users and self-caring public
• supports existing and promotes new arts and humanities therapies but also democratises this kind of approach
• diversifies beyond 'medical' to allied health and third sector involvement
• maximises the links between creativity, health and well-being
• contributes to the development of more compassionate environments for healthcare, health and well-being in hospitals and community or home settings
• promotes co-design, co-creativity and co-learning rather than an expert to lay approach.

The book calls for bringing the human back into health through the arts and humanities but not simply through a focus on developing the hearts and minds, even consultation and observational skills, of medical or allied health professionals. It expressly calls for a more extensive, mutual and applied field of work for delivering better social and cultural futures.

2
Anthropology and the Study of Culture

Anthropology and Cultural Studies

In this chapter we will consider the role of anthropology and the study of culture in the health humanities. Whilst there is a long tradition of medical anthropology – a field which has its own journals and many books – the relationship between this and the humanities has been less frequently thought about in a systematic way. Anthropology, as it has classically been thought of, is a comparative discipline concerned with patterns in human societies, in relation to cultural, social, psychological and biological dimensions. Belief systems, rituals, patterns of child rearing, family and kinship structure, language, ways of spending spare time, ways of making a living as well as the thorny topics of health and disease all play a part in anthropology. The field has a broad geographical and historical outlook. It deals not only with that small proportion of humankind in Europe and North America but with cultures and societies of the entire world. In its historic interests it can cover questions of human origins and our prehistoric past through to problems and dilemmas in the present day. It is also, along with philosophy, one of the oldest kinds of human inquiry. The intellectuals of classical antiquity puzzled over the differences and similarities between groups of people, and in the present day anthropology has contributed to disciplines as diverse as cognitive science, forensics, studies of diversity and ethnicity, linguistics and evolutionary studies. As a result of the pioneering work of individuals such as Franz Boas (1858–1942), the rather crude reliance on theories of racial differences popular in the 19th century gave way to an insistence on the role of culture, and its central importance in understanding differences between groups of human beings. Boas also popularised a notion of equipoise or cultural relativism – that is, the view that anthropology should not start out from the position that one culture is better or more advanced than another. Rather, in this view, the task of anthropology was to understand how culture shaped people to conceptualise and interact with the world in different ways, by means of gaining an understanding of their language and cultural practices.

Anthropology has a long history of association with medicine. Indeed, it was one of the cornerstones of medical education in the 19th century, and it was only as medicine became more reliant on the laboratory sciences and large academic teaching hospitals in the late 19th century that anthropology began to play a less prominent role (McElroy and Townsend, 1989). Even so, a number of key contributors to anthropology have had medical backgrounds, including W. H. R. Rivers and Arthur Kleinman. Some of the most compelling accounts in the anthropological literature concern the conceptualisation of illness in different parts of the world and human responses to it. We shall consider some examples of this shortly. However, it is important to note that the role of culture in how we experience, think about and respond to health and illness is a pervasive one, and this applies close to home as well as in unfamiliar cultures.

The systematic study of cultural forms in the British Isles was given a major boost by the development of the discipline of cultural studies. The term itself originates in the study of cultural artefacts or texts. Its history is often traced to pioneering scholars such as Richard Hoggart and Stuart Hall. The origins of the field have been traced to the founding by Hoggart of the Centre for Contemporary Cultural Studies at Birmingham University in 1964. Cultural studies drew upon the humanities but redefined the subject matter to include a whole variety of topics not usually studied by humanities scholars up to that point. Popular film and television, girls' magazines, popular music and youth subcultures, young people in the education system, policy and media discourse about social problems such as crime and 'race' – all these came within the ambit of this new field. The techniques of textual and linguistic analysis, contributions from psychoanalysis, critical social theory and Marxism were all added into the mix and used to explore these and many other aspects of culture.

As well as a focus on forms of social organisation and cultural behaviour, and patterns of linguistic and non-linguistic communication, cultural studies brings with it a scepticism about individual experience derived from European philosophy and social theory. Whereas the humanistic tradition in the health humanities has set a great deal of store by personal experience and first-hand narratives, cultural studies often seeks to decompose these and show how, for example, the notion of an individual, a person, or an 'authentic' experience are just as much social constructions as the organisations and relationships in which they occur. A focus on how the person exists within systems of ideology has highlighted how the interior world is informed by systems of ideology, language and social practice, and the focus on gender, race and social class has highlighted that there are often conflicts and tensions in cultural life, which may be played out in our relationship with one another, with journalism, popular magazines, films and drama, and the education system. From this perspective all forms of culture are interesting and worthy of study – not just the canonical high culture of the arts but the more mundane ways in which we might flick through a magazine, watch television or take a headache pill. There is culture at all points.

Anthropology, Culture and Illness

Throughout a good deal of western intellectual history illness has been seen to be about the body, and has been grounded in the physiology of the person. Yet even this formulation of the issue is a cultural construction in at least part. After all, the majority of the world's human civilisations past and present have not subscribed to this view. The value of a grasp of culture can be appreciated especially when we consider how particular health problems have arisen or new disease categories originated.

The relationship between anthropological study and health is often illustrated in Europe and North America by reference to seemingly exotic illnesses and healing practices from unfamiliar cultures. Examples which regularly appear in this context include *koro*, where the sufferer believes his or her genitals are shrinking or disappearing. It has been reported in China, Malaysia and Africa among other places (Dzokkoto and Adams, 2005; Mattelaer and Jilek, 2007). Another example is provided by the condition of *zou huo ru mo* which is sometimes found in China or among people of Chinese ancestry elsewhere in the world (Shan, 2000). This is a psychological and physiological disorder, involving the perception that there is an uncontrolled flow of 'qi' or life energy in the body. It may involve localised aches and pains, headaches, difficulties in falling asleep and even uncontrolled spontaneous movements. The intriguing thing about this condition is that it ties in with a variety of aspects of the beliefs and world-views of people in the region. It is believed by sufferers to indicate that something has gone awry with *qigong*, or the practice of cultivating 'life energy'. Yet another example is found among African students striving for success, who may be susceptible to brain fag syndrome. This involves bodily symptoms, including pains in the head, neck and eyes, difficulties with sleep, as well as cognitive impairment including difficulty in concentrating and retaining information (Ola et al., 2009).

These kinds of terms, experiences and clusters of symptoms might seem unusual to those familiar with Western healthcare. Accordingly, anthropologists and psychiatrists often use the term 'culture-bound syndrome' to denote a disorder which is specific to, and recognisable within, a specific culture (Guarnaccia and Rogler, 1999). Similarly, within its *Diagnostic and Statistical Manual* the American Psychiatric Association describes what it calls 'localized, folk, diagnostic categories that frame coherent meanings for certain repetitive, patterned, and troubling sets of experiences and observations' (American Psychiatric Association, 1994, p. 844).

In these cases anthropologists tend to emphasise the unique or culturally specific elements, but often physicians seek to identify parallels with well-known syndromes in Western psychiatry. For example, *zou huo ru mo*, with its unusual beliefs about the body and its workings, is sometimes seen as being akin to psychosis. In similar vein, culture-bound syndromes are often said to represent a locally intelligible or acceptable way within a specific culture to express distress in the wake of a traumatic experience among certain vulnerable individuals, and provides relatives, onlookers and local healers with a way of making sense of what seems to be unusual or bizarre behaviour.

The discipline of anthropology also encourages us to think more holistically about the nature of the societies in which particular phenomena and experiences occur. An example of the interplay of possession experiences with national, religious and gender identity as well as new technologies and ways of working is provided in a classic study by Aihwa Ong (1987). In her work *Spirits of Resistance* she described how life has changed for people in Malaysia in the late 20th century with the development of the electronics industry. In this predominantly Muslim area the electronics industry has provided a great deal of work for young women, who were consequently deferring marriage and providing an income for their families by seeking employment within it. The women were therefore released from some traditional forms of familial authority yet subject to some new forms of workplace discipline. Yet all did not run smoothly for the women or the factory proprietors:

> In 1975 forty Malay operators were seized by spirits in a large American electronics plant based in Sungai Way. A second large-scale incident in 1978 involved some 120 operators ... the factory had to be shut down for three days and a spirit healer was hired to slaughter a goat on the premises. (Ong, 1987, p. 204)

In a sense, these experiences of spirit possession and the disruption they caused contain a critical message that had otherwise been neglected by the industrial occupiers of Malaysian territory. In one American factory described by Ong (1987, p. 204):

> Some girls started sobbing and screaming hysterically and when it seemed like spreading, the other workers in the production line were immediately ushered out.... It is a common belief among workers that the factory is 'dirty' and supposed to be haunted by a *datuk*.

Whilst village elders and employees (especially newer ones) favoured explanations based on spirit possession and haunting, managers often took a more prosaic approach. They attributed some of these episodes to things like hunger from starting work early with no breakfast or the upheaval of changing from rural life to factory work. The measures they took against this included inviting local religious leaders to visit the factory and pray and perform rituals with holy water when new buildings were opened. Ong, on the other hand, sees the manifestations of possession as to do with a kind of resistance workers were showing to the dominance of multinational electronics firms and the way their lives were changing under these new economic conditions. As she puts it:

> Caught up in the problematics of labour and the problematics of self, resistance within the institutional constraints of capitalist production called forth images of social dislocation, draining of their essence, and violation of their humanity. (Ong, 1987, p. 220)

The spirit possessions therefore were, as she puts it in her title, spirits of resistance. This is similar to what Michael Taussig (1977) had argued a decade before in his account of peasant workers who tended to see representatives of capitalism and its way of doing things as being permeated with evil. This, says Taussig, represented a mode of critique of capitalist relations on the part of Colombian plantation workers.

Sometimes then, as with the work of Ong and Taussig, by taking this holistic view it is possible to see parallels between religious experiences, spirit possessions and the sense of evil and people's unhappiness with what is happening to them and their communities.

Spirit Possession

Reading accounts of unusual ailments and spirit possessions it often appears that these are characteristic of far-away places out of reach of Western medicine. Certainly, this has been attractive territory in anthropology where the study of cultures and societies unlike those of Western Europe and North America has taken priority. In some of the classic work on the anthropology of spirit possession it is clear that there are marked differences in the prevalence of this phenomenon. The frequency of such experiences is particularly variable. In some communities that hold possession beliefs, only a small percentage of the population is ever affected. For example, Wijesinghe et al. (1976) reported an incidence of 0.5 per cent for a community in Sri Lanka; Carstairs and Kapur (1976) found a period prevalence rate in a rural population on the west coast of South India of 2.8 per cent; and Venkataramaiah et al. (1981) reported a prevalence of 3.7 per cent in a different South Indian rural population. In other societies, the rates of possession are extremely high. For instance, in the villages of the Malagasy speakers of Mayotte, Lambek (1980) reported that 39 per cent of the adult women and 8 per cent of the adult men were considered to be possessed. Similarly, Harper (1963) reported that 20 per cent of the women among the Havik Brahmins in Mysore, India, experienced possession, and Boddy (1988) found between 42 and 47 per cent of married women over the age of 15 in the village of Hofriyat in Sudan had experienced possession. Considering only women of between 35 and 55 years, Boddy (1988) discovered that 66.6 per cent had suffered possession.

Although a community where around half of the population appear to have suffered some sort of spirit or demonic possession might seem rather unusual, it is instructive to think about what parallels we can see with so-called developed nations. With mental health problems specifically, it is not unusual to hear both professionals and lay people talking about disorders as if they had personalities of their own. When a person's untoward actions are attributed to their depression, their attention deficit hyperactivity disorder, or more colloquially, their 'hormones' or their 'nerves', a similar process is at work in making sense of ourselves, albeit one more in line with the scientific spirit of the day.

Even though possession experiences might seem exotic, the kinds of phenomena we have described are also apparent in the United States. Ross et al. (2013) explore dissociative experiences, which they, like many other authors, see as typically sudden, time-limited alterations in identity, behaviour and mental state. These are widely believed to be akin to experiences of possession in the literature on transcultural psychiatry (Bourguignon, 1976; Cardeña et al., 2009; Huskinson, 2010; Krippner, 1997; Lewis-Fernandez, 1994; Suryani and Jensen, 1993; Swartz, 2011). Ross et al.'s own participants, recruited from a programme for traumatised individuals in the United States, reported a great many dissociative experiences, that is, involving a sense of detachment from reality, and, interestingly, reported involvement in a wide range of healing rituals other than conventional medicine. Participants described how they had undergone a number of different exorcism procedures and shamanistic rituals (Eliade, 1964), including the feeling of having objects sucked out of their bodies, having their healer undergo a trance state during a ritual, engaging in activities intended to retrieve their soul, ritual dancing, animal sacrifice and being washed with blood.

Therefore it is entirely possible for healing practices that are at odds with Western medicine to co-exist with it. Ross et al.'s findings imply that similar social, cultural and psychological forces operate in the United States as they do in many other parts of the world. Furthermore Ross et al.'s data suggest that to an independent observer, English-speaking Caucasian Americans are just as capable of exhibiting these 'culture-bound syndromes' as any other group in the world. Indeed, beyond Ross et al.'s study, in everyday life it is not unusual to find people drawing on a variety of different healing regimes and belief systems at the same time. They may be obtaining prescribed medication via their general practitioner, may be seeking counselling, taking any of a range of widely available complementary and alternative remedies, seeking spiritual comfort via established religions or new age practitioners, and having acupuncture.

Close study of the findings of Ross et al., or studies like it, also enables us to think rather more critically about everyday statements that are commonly made about cross-cultural differences in consciousness: 'Oh, hearing voices is considered fairly normal in the such-and-such tribe'. Well, not necessarily. As Ross et al. show, participants' symptoms did not occur solely as part of an accepted religious practice. They were recognised as anomalous in the different faith communities of which they were members too. The symptoms were typified as pathological, and that was why the non-medical practitioners addressed them with a variety of shamanistic and religious methods 'usually thought of as primitive and culture bound' (Ross et al., 2013, p. 232).

Histories and Genealogies of Illness

Examining the history or genealogy of illnesses, disorders and complaints is often instructive too. This can give valuable information about the context and the enabling conditions relating to a particular problem. A fascinating example is provided by Hillel Schwartz (1989), who discusses the emergence of the idea of kleptomania, a compulsion to steal, in medico-legal discourse in the 19th century. This, he remarked, appeared with the development of department stores in major American and European cities, which were considered suitable places for middle class women to spend their time recreationally browsing and shopping. It was noted that many women who availed themselves of the opportunities to browse these new stores were accused of stealing from among the attractively displayed merchandise. Most puzzlingly, they stole items which they could easily have paid for and were not of any obvious necessity. At the time punishments for theft in many of the world's major judicial systems were harsh and often involved hard labour. Accordingly, the notion of kleptomania soon emerged to address this difficulty. As Schwartz documents, there were a number of explanations proffered, for example that the woman's inner child had got the better of her, or that she had been overcome by the sensuous attraction to the commodity and was therefore compelled to steal. Here is one example described by Schwartz:

> The sentence against a French woman convicted in 1844 of three petty thefts was overturned when a physician showed that the woman's entire character changed when she was stealing gloves, ribbons, cloth, brooches: normally, she was a calm, reasonable economical housewife and mother, but when she was in the kleptomaniac state, she was agitated, bitter, profligate, and a lover of vegetable soups. (Schwartz, 1989, p. 413)

At the time, in a curious parallel with the present day, some commentators saw this tendency as a sign of the times, as suggesting the adverse effects of commodity displays and one of the untoward effects of capitalism. What is interesting from our point of view is that particular economic and social developments, such as new ways of shopping, enabled the spaces into which new forms of experience, and new kinds of illness, could unfold. If one were a member of the lower classes and stole as a result of hunger, this could, almost by definition, not be kleptomania, and would be punished accordingly. Being conscious of one's needs meant that one was in control of one's faculties and could not be stealing as a result of an illness.

The relationship between the overall circumstances of a society and how its members conceptualise what ails them can be seen nearer the present too, as well as in the past. The way people described the experience of health and illness in a Mexican community studied by Castro (1995) was intimately bound up with their social circumstances. To the impoverished inhabitants of Ocuituco, the terms used to describe illness and wellness relate to material circumstances.

To be healthy is to be *gordo*, which means fat, fleshy or stout. To be ill is to be *flaco*, which means thin. Health, then, is conceptualised as fat, with the implication that one is having enough to eat.

The focus on the history of a condition can also be illuminating if one considers it in relation not only to the history of beliefs in a community but also the recent political history through which people and communities have lived. Devon Hinton and his colleagues (Hinton et al., 2013) have worked a great deal with Cambodians suffering something akin to post-traumatic stress disorder after the Pol Pot period. What he discovered was that this group possesses a unique 'bereavement ontology' in which dreams of the dead play a crucial role. As Hinton et al. explain:

> Encountering a dead person's spirit in a dream reveals that that person has not yet attained rebirth. When a friend or relative dies, patients carefully attend to such dreams and family members share these dreams to exchange information about the spiritual status of the deceased. (Hinton et al., 2013, p. 434)

Dying suddenly as a result of violence, or even in a road accident, is considered to be a 'bad death'. In the local belief system, which emphasises reincarnation, a bad death may indicate that a person has committed some kind of offence in a previous life. Moreover, a person who had died in the conflict in Cambodia would not have had relatives to hand to perform the rituals which are believed necessary to speed their path to their next life. Also, especially as families were split up by the Khmer Rouge, it is believed that the dead themselves cannot make progress because they miss their loved ones and therefore cannot make the transition to their next life. Seeing a deceased relative in a dream means that their soul is still wandering the earth and has not moved on to another life. Therefore dreaming of deceased people plays an important part in the experience of bereavement. One woman described by Hinton et al. recalled dreams in which her late father asked her why she had not been making offerings at the temple on his behalf. A young man whose family had been abused and executed by Khmer Rouge loyalists dreamed of his father being tortured. It has been suggested to him by a monk that this meant his father missed him and that it would be appropriate to undertake rituals in order to increase his late father's spiritual capital.

The man did so and this formed an important part of his coming to terms with the experience. These rituals – making offerings at temples and burning incense for example – undertaken in response to the dreams and recollections helped mitigate the painfulness of the experience and helped relieve the crying, multiple somatic symptoms, and flashback incidents.

This example indicates therefore that anthropological understanding of people's beliefs, conduct and the meanings particular communities attach to experiences can be valuable in making sense of what is happening. It is also valuable in placing into perspective and context what categories of illness and disorder themselves mean. Arthur Kleinman (1988a) coined the term 'category fallacy' to describe the problems in applying a category such as depression to different cultures when its characteristics in the West do not fully match that cultural context. Hinton et al. (2013) prefer the term 'category truncation' to describe the way key aspects of phenomena in a specific cultural context are left out of evaluation and criteria developed in Europe and the United States. As Hinton et al. observe, there is not always 'content equivalence' in the symptoms of bereavement or post-traumatic stress related disorder in different nations or cultures. For bereaved people it may be that some emphasise bodily symptoms, whereas others highlight depression and others still may focus on spiritual dimensions. Indeed, certain symptoms may be unique to a particular culture, or even a neighbourhood or community.

Ritual

A further insight from anthropology that is of particular value from the point of view of making sense of health and developing new approaches to treatment and therapy is that of ritual. The importance of this is alluded to in our discussion of Hinton's work in Cambodia above, and it is worth exploring the value of the study of ritual phenomena in more detail. Turner (1969), an anthropologist who made a major contribution to ritual studies, defined ritual as 'a stereotyped sequence of activities involving gestures, words, and objects, performed in a sequestered place and designed to influence preternatural [magical] entities or forces on behalf of the actors' goals and interests' (p. 18). Rituals are often found marking points of transition – developmental gateways in the lives of individuals. Ritual may help maintain group solidarity and equilibrium and provide a sense of control over fate and destiny. Rituals may also yield a protected time and space for the safe, cathartic discharge of intense emotions and promote emotional and physical healing (Bell, 1997; Csordas, 1987; Driver, 1998; Koss-Chioino, 2006; Malinowski, 1997; Turner, 1969; van Gennep, 1960; Wallace, 1966). DeFlem (1991, p. 3) claims that whilst rituals can involve performances, rituals themselves are transformational activities and that 'the handling of symbols in ritual exposes their powers to act upon and change the persons involved in ritual performance'.

Turner (1969) and van Gennep (1960) have argued that ritual becomes especially prominent at times of uncertainty, anxiety and disorder because rituals dramatise messages of continuity, predictability and tradition. In this view rituals appear to have a stabilising influence and serve to integrate the self with itself, particularly in the face of social change. Rituals help to define and reinforce the relationship of the self with culture via the sharing of common experiences, symbols, language, objects and performances. Rituals are also significant in shaping and managing the relationship between the self and others (communitas), and the self in relation to divine or natural forces which are believed to influence the future.

The concepts of death and dying, and the activities surrounding these, involve a particularly rich and widely studied area of anthropological and ritual interest. Individuals from many cultures have particular views on how this might be accomplished auspiciously – from ideas about places and times to die to views on how surviving relatives should best organise funeral rituals through to ideas about what will happen to the deceased afterwards, human cultures have been particularly rich in this regard. The stories told, and the way that these experiences are made meaningful, represent valuable resources through which the scholar or practitioner can gain insight, build relationships and engage in culturally sensitive practice in this field.

For example, Venkatasalu et al. (2014) describe a study in which they interviewed people of South Asian origin living in London about their expectations and aspirations surrounding dying. One feature that stood out clearly was that people often wished to go back to what they saw to be their home country to die.

Kamruz: Yes. I would like to die in Bangladesh. May God prove my
wish? Definitely I love to die on my own Bangladeshi soil. Yes I am
British. This is my country as well. But I was born in Bangladesh.
I came to this country during my adulthood. I adopted this coun-
try, I love this country as well, but for my death, my own village
will be the best place to die.
M.R.V.: Could you tell me more?
Kamruz: Because I was born there. I want to die there. Because
that will be more comfortable than dying here actually. (Kamruz,
Bangladeshi male, age 58 years) (Venkatasalu et al., 2014, p. 267)

This sense of connection with a homeland, whilst commonplace in
Venkatasalu et al.'s study, was not the only orientation. Some who
had been born in the UK did not have so strong a sense of attachment overseas, and others said that their former friends and relatives
in the family's country of origin would be dispersed and no longer
available. For others, the key issue was whether they could expect
the appropriate companionship and ritual as they died. An elderly
woman from Kerala said:

I want someone to be near me so they can pray. But it won't
happen if we die in hospital. I would prefer to have my children
with me, and if that's not possible, then I at least want to be with
someone that I can trust if I am conscious. (Venkatasalu et al.,
2014, p. 268)

This often yielded a preference for dying at home rather than in hospital, in the company of family members, so the rituals and prayers
could be performed in a way which they saw to be appropriate. This
was seen as important in achieving a peaceful and dignified death and
a way of enabling family members to do their duty to one another. It
is through this anthropological understanding of ritual and through
an awareness of the role it plays in people's lives that services can be
adapted most effectively to different communities' needs.

Very often when we think of ritual, it is tempting to imagine practices which are ancient and have remained more or less unchanged
for hundreds of years. However, rituals are living practices and are
frequently adapted to new circumstances, opportunities and con-
straints. Equally, sometimes new rituals are created to help address

new experiences. For example, over the last half century a variety of agencies, therapists, justice professionals, public service bodies and women themselves have changed dramatically the way they recognise and attempt to address domestic violence. Where survivors of these experiences are concerned, a number of therapeutic approaches have been employed. Of particular interest from the point of view of this chapter is an approach described by Allen and Wozniak (2014), who report an initiative based around ritual for women who were seeking to come to terms with and move on from experiences of domestic violence. In a groupwork setting they engaged in a variety of discussions and rituals such as the following:

> [A] 'power mantra' activity in which women read together this affirmation: *I reclaim my power from all those who have tried to take it. I reclaim my power from the universe that held it for me until this moment. I reclaim my power and will never let it go again. I feel my power re-enter my body, mind and spirit. I am filled with the power of love and joy.* Women then created a personal gesture that accompanied the mantra. This gesture would be used as a sign for each woman and for her group mates indicating that she had embraced and reclaimed her own power. (Allen and Wozniak, 2014, p. 60)

In addition to these communal activities and the value they had for participants, Allen and Wozniak were in a position to examine how ritual was invented. When 'ritual emerged, it was quickly codified, ritualized, and incorporated into the regular, predictive patterns of group behaviour that were endowed with meaning and value by group participants' (Allen and Wozniak, 2014, p. 57). This has parallels with the kinds of strategies used to combat negative statements about the self that can be found in cognitive behavioural therapy. Yet it is also something that draws on more primordial traditions of magic. Rituals may be effective, as Kwan (2007) suggests, through their 'dynamic, diachronic, and physical characteristics. In other words, ritual efficacy lies in the manner of performance; not in any rational discursive argument' (p. 747).

The idea of ritual makes an interesting analytical lens with which to view a good deal of healthcare practice. The activities involved in suffering and healing, the gifts and exchanges in healthcare rituals, the sights, sounds and smells, the elaborate dance of practitioner and client can all be seen as a kind of ritual. In this way we can begin to understand that applying a sticking plaster to a minor injury, getting a prescription at the end of a consultation with a doctor or having one's chest listened to with a stethoscope are freighted with meaning far beyond the physical characteristics of the intervention or assessment.

To take a slightly more involved empirical example of this approach to understanding the practice of healthcare, let us consider an account by Tjørnhøj-Thomsen and Hansen (2013) of a residential rehabilitation programme for cancer survivors in Denmark. The programme in question consisted of a weeklong stay in a converted castle, with a variety of group and individual activities intended to address patients' informational needs and psychosocial issues. In some cases the staff running the programme deliberately invoked make believe. For example, as part of the introduction 'participants were told that this week they would be the "ladies (or lords) of the manor" and that the castle "belonged to them." The temporary and illusory transfer of co-ownership to the castle conjured up an image of nobleness, an image that strengthened the participants' feelings of being special and cared for' (Tjørnhøj-Thomsen and Hansen, 2013, p. 271).

Turner (1974) notes that ritual has a capacity to transcend and transform familiar social roles, structures and boundaries. This reversal of structure is something that he terms 'antistructure', which can be viewed as a temporary suspension of the requirements of everyday norms and roles that provide a critical distance from structure and social-structural norms (Turner, 1974, pp. 42–43). Thus in the programme studied by Tjørnhøj and Hansen, some of the roles and power structures usually associated with the practice of medicine were subverted and inverted. 'We (the staff) are the experts in the disease, but you (the participants) are the experts in your situation.' The staff stated that they wanted to 'learn from the participants' (p. 272). The caring attentiveness of the staff left a deep impression on the participants, and formed a sharp contrast to the participants' treatment experiences elsewhere in the healthcare system, such as feelings of being a number and not a human being, of not being listened to or taken seriously (cf. Sered, 1999). The programme participants' experiences of being cared for and listened to by the staff formed part of a re-humanising process. Care and attentiveness from the staff generated a sense for the participants of being recognised as human beings again after a long journey through treatment in the medical system. Like rituals studied by anthropologists, this process helped facilitate a change in status towards a new socially defined self; a process of 'strategic socialisation' (Bell, 1992). However, unlike the rituals studied in so-called 'tribal' societies, the clients' journeys beyond the rehabilitation programme tended to be individual ones where they took on individual responsibility for managing their illness and its after-effects. Nevertheless, as Seligman (2010, p. 15) suggests,

> [...] through its emphasis on action, on the performative and its creation of a subjunctive universe, ritual creates a world, temporary, fragile to be sure, but not false – a world where differences can be accommodated, tolerance enacted (if not fully understood) and openness to the other maintained.

A subjunctive universe, that is one which emphasises counterfactuals, possibilities and imaginings of things that may yet come true, is often specifically invited by ritual. In that way, the ideas invited by a make believe, counterfactual world can facilitate progress:

> It has always been the prime function of mythology and rite to supply the symbols that carry the human spirit forward, in counteraction to those other constant human fantasies that tend to tie it back. (Campbell, 1949, p. 11)

Rituals then have a paradoxical function. They provide some of the glue that holds social conventions together, and they also provide the possibility of change. In this way, in both so-called 'traditional' societies and in late modernity they have important roles to fulfil, and looking at healthcare through the lens of ritual can yield a great deal of insight for heath humanities.

Summary and Conclusions

Summing up the value of an anthropological and cultural perspective on healthcare, Lambert and McKevitt (2002) indicated how anthropology applied to medicine can assist medicine in viewing familiar phenomena afresh, reconceptualise a problem's boundaries and hence yield novel insights. Anthropology emphasises the value of data gathered informally, the difference between what people say and what they do, and critically examining not just 'lay' beliefs but professional knowledge too.

But there is much still to be done. Whilst a good deal of cross-cultural study in healthcare has focused on mental health, with illuminating results, physical illnesses have received far less scrutiny of this kind. Anthropologists have tended to side with their medical colleagues and left many of the illness categories of Western medicine undisturbed by their unwillingness to engage critically with the biological sciences. These disciplines have cultures of their own and construct knowledge and belief systems which are then disseminated through the social fabric. This kind of framing of the human body and its workings is as susceptible to anthropological interrogation as any other belief system.

As Hemmings (2005) points out, the healthcare disciplines need anthropology, because the benefits of healthcare are not being delivered efficiently. Hemmings contends that much greater progress would be made in medicine if existing treatments were effectively used. Healthcare practitioners are often not well aware of the evidence concerning lay beliefs and practices, and health education programmes often fail through misunderstanding their audience.

In this respect perhaps the final thought should be from anthropologist and psychiatrist Arthur Kleinman who nearly four decades ago pointed to the importance of examining people's own explanatory models about their health. This approach brings together the anthropological and clinical modes of inquiry:

> Eliciting the patient's (explanatory) model gives the physician knowledge of the beliefs the patient holds about his illness, the personal and social meaning he attaches to his disorder, his expectations about what will happen to him and what the doctor will do, and his own therapeutic goals. Comparison of patient model with the doctor's model enables the clinician to identify major discrepancies that may cause problems for clinical management. Such comparisons also help the clinician know which aspects of his explanatory model need clearer exposition to patients (and families), and what sort of patient education is most appropriate. And they clarify conflicts not related to different levels of

knowledge but different values and interests. Part of the clinical process involves negotiations between these explanatory models, once they have been made explicit. (Kleinman et al., 1978, p. 255)

This concern, if it is followed through into anthropological or clinical practice, leads to a set of questions that may be deployed. These, following Kleinman, may look something like the following:

- What do you think has caused your problem?
- Why do you think it started when it did?
- What do you think your sickness does to you? How does it work?
- How severe is your sickness? Will it have a short or long course?
- What kind of treatment do you think you should receive?
- What are the most important results you hope to receive from this treatment?
- What are the chief problems your sickness has caused for you?
- What do you fear most about your sickness?

It is through questions like these that practitioners in the health humanities can borrow productively from anthropological traditions of inquiry and see how the participant, client or anyone else frames the problem in their own terms and what they are seeking by way of treatment or remedy. In this way the anthropological outlook can make a significant contribution to the value of the humanities in health.

3
Applied Literature

Health humanities, from its valuable inception and discoursal development as the medical humanities through to its evolution into a 'more inclusive and applied approach to humanities in healthcare', engages not only scholars and medics but all forms of 'practitioners, healthcare providers, patients and their carers' (Crawford et al., 2010, p. 8) and has a long and varied engagement with literature, in the broadest sense of all forms of written text (Charon, 2000). Concern with literature, writing or text, and health and illness, can be seen in a multitude of intersecting functional and academic endeavours, from the use of literature in the education of doctors (Evans, 2003), to the development of medically-focused scholarly or literary analysis of specific texts and conditions or traumas (such as epilepsy in literature – Jones, 2000; or the psychological impact of rape in Angela Carter's fiction – Baker, 2011) and the therapeutic uses of constructing narrative (Baikie and Wilhelm, 2005; Crawford et al., 2004; Ross, 2012). Literature – both fiction in a range of forms and autobiographical narratives, including pathographies – can tell us not only about medicine or doctors, but also about the experience of health, sickness, illness, encounters with clinics and clinicians, the reactions of significant others, the support found in the strangest of places, the role and impact of informal caring, and the radical reordering necessary after the dramatic rift that significant illness causes through an individual life. This chapter focuses on three core areas of the intersection of literature and health. Firstly, in the opening section, some considerations are provided on the literary genre of *pathography* – illness in literature – with a particular focus on madness or mental health challenges as they are portrayed in fiction. The second section discusses the value and use of stories in clinical education, practice and research. Finally, some brief tentative observations around the therapeutic value of reading will be given.

Illness, Health and Sickness in Literature

All of us have stories to tell, and we tell stories every day. We recount, relate, reflect, revise and re-evaluate ourselves and our experiences via narratives – narratives we tell ourselves and those that we choose to share (Frank, 1995, p. 53). As a range of scholars who have explored illness narratives attest, experiencing any form of illness that requires medium- or long-term adjustments, causes disability, challenges the sense of personhood, or forces an encounter with the possibility of death, tests our capacity to not only survive and to live well, but to readjust our futures, sense of self, aims and goals. A few days in bed with a cold or a sprained ankle of course generally does not require such radical reassessment, though a disappointment may occur if the injury or illness results in missing a crucial event or exam, for example. Longer-term or life-threatening conditions – from diabetes or asthma, requiring daily medication, through to chronically painful conditions such as Crohn's disease or arthritis, or those conditions that are widely misunderstood like endometriosis or schizophrenia, or the most feared of illnesses – cancer – or the diagnoses which fundamentally will change the self as coherent being, such as dementia all challenge individuals in different ways. Illnesses sit along a spectrum between health and death, all to varying degrees, leaving the individual potentially in a liminal state of flux and uncertainty, pain and hesitation, fear and anxiety. At these times, an acute need to bring order and understanding to the chaotic challenge, or to have others validate the experience of crisis, can be felt. At these times, stories emerge from us in emotive, painful and graphic ways.

Unsurprisingly then, perhaps, the most obvious encounter of literature and medicine lies in the literary genre of pathography. Anne Whitehead, providing an insightful critical and historical overview of the origins of literary-focused medical humanities that have developed in the UK and US, suggests that for 'both writer and reader [...] pathography functions as the site of a limit experience, an encounter

with (possible) death that engages powerful questions of consciousness, agency, and identity' (Whitehead, 2014, p. 113). Pathography –
the writing of the illness experience – has a long and diverse history,
of interest not only to scholars in literature and clinicians but also
of course to those who have suffered and suffered with individuals
themselves.

Anne Hunsaker Hawkins (1993, 1999) and Arthur Frank (1995)
have provided useful typographies of pathographic narrative.
Hawkins suggests that pathography – which she defines as 'a form
of autobiography or biography that describes personal experiences
of illness, treatment, and sometimes death' (1993, p. 1) – can be best
seen as a '*re*-formulation of the experience of illness':

> [...] as the artistic product and continuation of the instinctive
> psychological act of formulation: it gathers together the separate
> meanings, the moments of illumination and understanding, the
> cycles of hope and despair, and weaves them into a whole fabric,
> one wherein a temporal sequence of events takes on narrative
> form. (1993, pp. 24–25)

The 'task' of the author of the pathography is not only, as Hawkins
suggests, to 'describe this disordering process' but to 'restore to reality its lost coherence and to rediscover, or create, a meaning that can
bind it together again' (1993, pp. 2–3). Hawkins convincingly divides
pathographies into three main groups – testimonial pathography,
angry pathography and pathographies 'advocating alternative modes
of treatment' (1993, p. 4). These three types contain four 'mythic paradigms – battle, journey, rebirth and "healthy-mindedness"' (1993,
p. 28). Examining the surge in publication of these three subtypes
of autobiography over the past 50 years, she suggests that pathography functions not only as meaning-making in an individual sense,
but also in terms of restoring the *person* 'ignored or canceled out
in the medical enterprise', giving voice to experience (1993, p. 12).
Addressing inevitable concerns about the truth-value of pathography (like any form of retrospective creation, it will be subject to
retrograde sense-making, reordering and remembering), she suggests
that this act of re-creation is in itself valuable as it exposes the 'metaphoric and mythic constructs' about illness in a particular time and
culture (Hawkins, 1993, pp. 14–18 – see also pp. 25–26). Hawkins

closes with a useful bibliography of physical illness pathographies, particularly those concerned with cancer.

Similarly, Arthur Frank provides a detailed perspective on illness narratives, concentrating on the ethical imperative of both author and reader to understand the radical challenge to the self that bodily dysfunction poses. Frank focuses on three narrative types in his analysis – the restitution narrative, the chaos narrative, and the quest narrative. He suggests, like Hawkins, that illness narratives serve in many ways to restore a voice lost with a medical focus on the (sometimes disembodied) body, to re-establish a self through and beyond a limit experience dominated by medical discourse that focuses on a bodily ill (1995, pp. xii–xiii). For Frank, even 'edited stories remain true' – that is, the 'truth of stories is not only what *was* experienced, but equally what *becomes* experience in the telling and its reception' (p. 22). He argues throughout his work that stories of illness function as both a way of reorienting after a disordering or disorienting experience, and as recording that same significant experience (p. 53). Self-coherence and life-coherence can be 'restored' in the act of writing the illness experience (p. 61). The three types of narrative have different aims and effects, but all are important. The restitution narrative focuses on the journey through illness back to health. Conversely, the chaos narrative, less preferred in our cultural space where health is always a state to be not only restored to by medicine but to be sought after by the stoic sick person, focuses on the 'vulnerability, futility, and impotence' brought about through illness (p. 97). The quest narratives, however, 'meet suffering head on; they seek to *use* it' (p. 115). In this sense, different illnesses and different styles of management may lean people towards different narratological stances – the ordered re-telling, the inevitable but challenging immersion in the chaotic, or creation via the use-values of a 'limit' experience, as Whitehead refers to it (2014, p. 113). Frank closes with a focus on the testimonial value of illness narratives, and the moral and ethical purpose of reordering how such texts are received – instead of merely absorbing or taking something away from a story, both the writer and the reader must consider how a story (or stories) both endures *and* develops over time (1995, pp. 158–159). Frank's narrative types are discussed in more detail in Chapter 4.

Frank and Hawkins focus, in different ways, on the sense- or meaning-making value of pathography on both an individual and collective interpretative level. Critiquing the notion that sense-making or mastery over experience can be attained via writing, Whitehead suggests that rather 'than subscribing to a dominant impulse towards meaning and control' we might 'also benefit from what the literary can reveal to us about what it means to live in a condition of *uncer-tainty*' (2014, p. 115). She argues that a more 'expansive sense of the literary might, then, potentially also open up a more integrated approach to literature in the medical humanities; one which enables us to address medicine's own inherent uncertainties, and the skills of interpretative reading that it accordingly requires of its practitioners' (p. 115). Hence, it is not only the factual portrayal of (usually physical) illness experience – the personal depiction of pain or distortion, change or disability – that is, or should be, of interest within the health humanities. Fictional texts, which set in motion our interpretative capabilities in a different way, also have value in this sphere. As David Lodge says, 'literature is a record of human consciousness, the richest and most comprehensive we have [...] Works of literature describe in the guise of fiction the dense specificity of personal experience, which is always unique, because each of us has a slightly or very different personal history, modifying every new experience we have; and the creation of literary texts recapitulates this uniqueness' (2002, pp. 10–11). Fictional pathographies can thus also offer a mirror of the psychological and physical *experience* of sickness through their very construction – their textual creation, style, metaphoric chains, metonymic representation, languages and structures, charactorial creations – and the way we read fictional works can then in itself offer a space for reflection on the ways in which illness is encountered by us as either observers or experiencers.

Whether we focus on the uncertainty of resolution in a particular story as mirroring the experience of an uncertain diagnosis or choose to examine the not-good-patient elements of a created character, with their adjunct fears and uncertainty as telling us something about how it may feel to be anxious or afraid, fictional literary texts provide a diverse range of narratives of value to the health humanities. The interactional construction of dialogue in narratives may tell us something about the interpersonal encounter. Gendered exchanges that occur in the text may inform us about wider cultural issues relating to men, women and illnesses – the way in which a feminist analysis may look at how women are expected to respond passively to illness whereas men may be expected to be brave and battle, for example, or how exclusively female diseases like gynaecological cancers can be shrouded in mystery or shame. Other narratives, particularly those in the postmodern genre, may reveal something about the experience of postmodern existence, fragmented, fractured and chaotic, which circularly can inform us about the doubling of fragmentation that can occur if an already-fractured self experiences a further fracturing through an illness encounter (see Baker et al., 2010, chapter 6). We may choose to perform an analysis which closely follows those regularly enacted in literary studies, focusing on specific literary elements or readings, tropes or themes, style or linguistics (Eaglestone, 2009). At the least, a fictional text can transport us into another person's world for a short time, enabling both the vicarious and the banal to be equally sensed in a safe environment.

Madness in Literature

While much work on pathography has focused on the autobiographic tales of physical illness, the portrayal of madness in literature has attracted a significant amount of literary attention, almost forming a subgenre of its own in literary studies and contributing to a large body of academic work on fictional pathography, medicine in literature and charactorial study. Unlike a physical illness, the most extreme test of personal integrity and identity comes in the form of challenges to mental well-being, from depression and anxiety through to psychotic disorders which challenge not only the 'regular' experience of emotional health but the sense of secure and reliable perceptions and beliefs. It is unsurprising, perhaps, that madness – the threatened loss of selfhood, the turmoil of bleak emotions drawing a person towards a welcome death, the acute fear of an enigmatic agency monitoring a person's every move or threatening their safety, the guilt of an unspecific or perhaps minor past action overwhelming current life – has provided an assorted wealth of material for authors to draw from.

Literatures of madness both *tell* madness in their narrative themes but also *show* madness textually through deconstructed and destructed form, structure, internal dialogue and narration. Such literatures have a focus on that which is 'other'-than-sane, as Felman suggests:

> Society has built the walls of mental institutions to keep apart the inside and the outside of a culture, to separate between reason and unreason and to keep apart the other against whose apartness

society asserts its sameness and redefines itself as sane. But every literary text, I argue, communicates with madness – with what has been excluded, decreed abnormal, unacceptable, or senseless – by dramatizing a dynamically renewed, revitalized relation between sense and nonsense, between reason and unreason, between the readable and the unreadable. (1985, p. 5)

In this sense, it is not only *personal* madness that is told through literary narratives, but also forms of societal or cultural *otherness*, that which is 'excluded' or 'decreed abnormal'. This recognition can certainly be seen in feminist scholarship that has, importantly, used literature that focuses on madness to explore the historical and current subjugation of women socially, culturally, politically and interpersonally (see Chesler, 2005; Gilbert and Gubar, 2000; Showalter, 1987).

Branimir M. Rieger, in an illuminating selection of essays on aspects of 'literary madness', asks 'from what better source could one learn about madness, violence, murder, deceit, betrayal, lust, greed, loneliness and depression than in writers such as Sophocles, Aeschylus, Shakespeare, Dostoyevsky, Faulkner, Genet, Nabakov, Burroughs and Stephen King?' (Rieger, 1994, p. 5). Rieger is astute in his assertion that literature provides insights into the human condition that are unavailable in such richly comprehensive, and unique, form elsewhere, such as in the clinical vignette. A second scholar, Lillian Feder, in her 1980 historico-cultural study of literature from Dionysus and Shakespeare through to Sylvia Plath, suggests that in 'literature, as in daily life, madness is the perpetual amorphous threat within and the extreme of the unknown in fellow human beings' (p. 4). For Feder, a 'mad literary character must be approached on his own terms, through the verbal, dramatic, and narrative symbols that convey the unconscious processes he portrays and reveals' (p. 9). Whereas the vignette or case study, under the guise of presenting a narrative of a unique experience, portrays a madness experience under a homogenising diagnostic framework, the literary text instead presents the individual human specificity of cognition, emotion and internality in imaginative and unique form. This in turn reminds us that there is no 'typical' experience of madness, despite the homogenising tendency of the common diagnostic systems. Nosology denies the elements of human agency and autonomy that the literary text epitomises. Considering the core principles which we are suggesting health humanities rides on, what we can see here is a consideration of the notion of the *democratising* of mental health. Literary portrayals of madness are both inclusive *and* exclusive – they allow for a personalising of mental health, a multiplicity of personal and carer or 'other' perspectives on distress and disorder that do not rely on medical formulation of the experience, but instead provide examples of a more outward-facing, non-hierarchal, individualised interpretation and view. The diversity of Rieger and Feder's works adds a further layer of difference here – the first being the text, the second being the readings *of* madness literatures, each distinct, each true.

Other literary scholars have explored specific elements of psychopathology in characters, such as depression with obsessional features in *Hamlet* (Shaw, 2002), or more broadly in contemporary fiction and culture, such as Timothy Melley's (2000) or Patrick O'Donnell's studies of paranoia. O'Donnell interestingly suggests:

> Paranoia as manifested in contemporary narrative can be further considered as the multifarious contradiction of a postmodern condition in which the libidinal investment in mutability, in being utterly other, contests with an equally intense investment in the commodification of discrete identities: this contradiction pertains both to the formation of individual subjects and to the national and political bodies into which they are interpellated as collective subjects. (2000, p. 14)

The result of this tension between individual identity and the pressures of a collective consciousness is that paranoia no longer can be seen as 'the classic, universalized symptom of an individual pathological condition' but instead 'can be seen as symptomatic of a collective identity' (O'Donnell, 2000, p. 14). O'Donnell here follows a fundamental concern shared by many postmodern theorists, from Jean Baudrillard (1983) to Fredric Jameson (1991), that postmodernity is best encapsulated as being defined and experienced as psychosis. Angela Woods provides an excellent and detailed study into how versions and representations of schizophrenia come to be a metaphor for contemporary post-war life in the work of a range of latter 20th-century thinkers, including in the fiction of Bret Easton Ellis – extending her analysis through a range of fictions would be an interesting addition to the health humanities (Woods, 2011). Hence, it can be suggested that – as Felman, Melley and O'Donnell imply – literary works *on* madness tell us much about cultural and societal expectations, constructions, beliefs and values (medical, health and other), at a specific time, which construe some as 'mad' and some as 'not', as well as of the individual experience of psychological health and illness. This is certainly the theme that Louis Sass explored in much detail in his famous 1992 study *Madness and Modernism: Insanity in the Light of Modern Art, Literature and Thought.*

Evelyne Keitel, like Frank and Hawkins, provides a fascinating reading of what she calls *psychopathographies*, texts which focus on madness in a range of ways and which 'first appeal to but then undermine and ultimately frustrate the reading habits acquired from consuming contemporary literature' (1989, p. 14). In reading texts belonging to this very specific subgenre of madness fictions, Keitel suggests 'a vacuum is created in which the specific effect of psychopathographies can unfold' (1989, p. 14). *Psychopatho*graphical texts, for Keitel, are distinguishable from *patho*graphical texts by virtue of their effect on the reader – the reader is not distanced from the psychosis depicted but is instead drawn into the midst of the experience where '[r]eading about psychosis becomes a reading psychosis' (p. 118 – see also Baker et al., 2010, pp. 24–26). She suggests that psychopathographies 'deal with an area of experience which resists linguistic representation'; but, of course, the 'literary strategies whereby psychotic experience is communicated are not – or at least, are not all – marked by unfamiliarity and strangeness of the subject matter' as 'inaccessible material cannot be communicated in an unknown code' (p. 14). Instead, she suggests, 'psychopathographies rely for their effect on textual strategies which are in part taken over from their literary context, and on experiences with reading other contemporary texts' (p. 14). Keitel then develops a convincing theory of reader response focusing on different types of psychopathography, exploring the effect of each based on their familiarity and distance from usual conventions of reading and comprehension.

Keitel's work is interesting and can be further developed through exploration of the range of distinctly postmodern authors who have provided literary texts (it is challenging to think of these as *narratives* in a traditional sense) that demonstrate what is referred to elsewhere as the *psychoticisation* of textual form and content (Baker et al., 2010, p. 165). Diverting from Keitel's work, some postmodern authors, for example Kathy Acker, William S. Burroughs and Philip K. Dick, write 'inaccessible' material through *new* – rather than 'unknown' – textual codes and strategies, requiring attention to aid development of new interpretative skills. The distinctly postmodern *psychotic* texts differ from Keitel's psychopathographies in their distorted linguistic and narrative form, loss of linear narrative, and dislocation of context and content. Such authors explore the way in which individual existence has become fraught with incoherence and fragmentation, rather than portraying clinically definable psychosis as per diagnostic definition (see Baker et al., 2010, chapter 6). If we return to Felman, the reading function of this subgenre of psychopathographies, those *psychotic texts*, can be viewed in a clinically relevant way. Felman concludes: 'even though the discourse *on* madness is not a discourse *of* madness (it is not strictly speaking a mad discourse), nevertheless there still exists in these texts a *madness that speaks*, a madness that is acted out in language, but whose role no speaking subjects can assume' (1985, p. 252). But psychotic texts are neither *of* nor *on* madness. The 'madness that speaks' is written into the textual structure of erratic narration – and in such fictions the *subject* speaks *through* and *within* madness. Attention to the unfamiliar experience of unpacking and interpreting such texts can enable clinically relevant skills in not only *hearing* psychosis but in interpreting the diverse strands of thought, emotion and belief that are presented in a manner which may be unfamiliar if psychosis has not been experienced. The clinical value here may be 'only' to provide the reader with a sense of how it may feel to experience chaos or anxiety, through a second-hand medium. But it could be that *reading* psychotic texts can promote the development of novel interpretative and communicative skills around psychosis – in sensing nuances or themes amidst confusion, acknowledging fracturing of self or I, recognising and sense-making of strangeness. There is not space to more fully illuminate this notion here – indeed, this subject could usefully be subject to further scrutiny – but the clinical utility of literature has been represented in a range of different ways, and it is to this area of literature and health that this chapter now turns.

Literature in Healthcare Education and Practice

The portrayal of madness in fiction has begun to attract the attention of practising nurses and medics, who explore how, through literary analysis, characters who are portrayed as mentally ill can provide insights into the experience of madness that is both different from and complementary to that found in a clinical textbook (Clarke, 2009; Oyebode, 2009). Whether the focus be on Shakespeare's *Hamlet* or *King Lear*, or more contemporary texts such as Patrick McGrath's brilliant portrayal of paranoia and psychosis in *Spider* (1990), Jeffrey Eugenides' evocative and strange *The Virgin Suicides* (1993) on teenage suicide, or Michael Ignatieff's *Scar Tissue* (1994) on memory loss and the role of informal caring, literature can offer insights into the *experience of experiences* which may be unfamiliar to the reader. One reason for immersion in literature is the opportunity to see inside or encounter something different, peculiar, as escapism or to gain a sense of something new, to learn or to develop empathy. The recently founded Madness and Literature Network at the University of Nottingham provides a database of fiction and autobiography focusing on madness (www.madnessandliterature.org). A range of pathographic literature focuses on madness. Autobiographies such as William Styron's brilliant *Darkness Visible* (1990) and Elizabeth Wurtzel's *Prozac Nation* (1994) provide insight into the acuity of emotional pain suffered with severe depression. There are other narratives which are semi-fictionalised autobiographies, like Sylvia Plath's *The Bell Jar* (1963) and Janet Frame's *Faces in the Water* (1961), both of which feature prominently in clinically-focused works on psychopathography in fiction, and which explore retrospectively the experience of severe depression and psychosis. The following chapter also briefly explores pathographies in relation to cancer and other forms of narratives of illness and health.

More recently, the voices of people with direct lived experience of mental health challenges have become recognised as valid and important sources of knowledge about altered mental states and the experience of distress, fear, anxiety, elation and unusual experiences – such unique narratives have begun to be collated and published (Baker et al., 2013; Cordle et al., 2011; Grant et al., 2011, 2013; Read and Reynolds, 1996). However, such collections, while seen as important in some circles, are not required reading in the same way psychiatry textbooks are, demonstrating a privileging of so-called 'objective' knowledge of mental health and illness over unique and subjective accounts. Enduringly popular are collections of extended vignettes about 'patients' from the perspective of their doctor, representing a secondary re-telling of illness and therapy that maintains the powerful doctor and passive patient positioning (Sacks, 1985; Yalom, 1989). Gail A. Hornstein's more recent *Agnes's Jacket* combines a literary narrative, about the autobiographical text that psychiatric patient Agnes Richter wove into her jacket, with the stories and words of those who use peer support and self-defined recovery in mental health in a fascinating collection that could well revise this precarious and outdated balance in mental health care (Hornstein, 2012).

There is a wealth of scholarship into the use of literature and humanities in medical education and as part of ongoing continuing professional development (Beveridge, 2003; Evans, 2003; Greenhalgh and Hurwitz, 1998; Oyebode, 2009; Tischler, 2010). Beveridge outlines the benefits for psychiatry, suggesting that literature provides a more personalised and in-depth existential understanding of psychiatric illnesses than clinical textbooks, enhancing empathic skills and reactions (2003, p. 385). Yet the use of literature in clinical education is seen, at best, as a useful and pleasant addition – but not a vital element. Beveridge outlines the critical arguments against this addition, illuminating critiques such as the humanities being irrelevant to clinical practice and the obvious fact that reading literature *on* mental health is not 'a substitute for experience' (2003, p. 386). Stempsey also questions whether teaching humanities and philosophy automatically enhances the humanity and humane response of future clinicians (1999). In spite of such concerns, there is now a growing body of work on the value of a humanities-based element to the education of other health professionals such as nurses and a recognition, in the challenging times of austerity, of the need to think creatively about approaches to health and healthcare (Crawford and Baker, 2009; McKie and Gass, 2001; Slade et al., 2008).

Creative resources, in clinical education, can promote creative reflection – though as Whitehead cautions, rather 'than harnessing literature to an existing agenda, in which empathy is treated as yet another skill for doctors to master', we might also 'productively connect clinical diagnosis and literary reading as necessarily uncertain, yet essential, models of interpretative practice' (2014, p. 116). Indeed, across all spectrums of health service personnel, and in informal carers and support group settings – clinical diagnosis is a small part of clinical practice – literary reading can aid the development of skills not only in (empathic) communication and explanation, but also in interpreting the person's *own* way of narrating their experiences, symptoms, concerns and fears. People do not always tell stories in linear or coherent ways. The art of a mutually beneficial clinical encounter (even if the overall aims are divergent) is to pull together the strands of the story into a coherent whole, while simultaneously attending to those parts of the story that the person privileges that the clinician may not in their search for a specific diagnosis, plan of care, risk assessment or symptom checking.

Two core pedagogic functions can be seen in using literature in clinical education. Literature – particularly first person accounts of illness, but also fiction, poetry, prose and reflective pieces from others – promotes the consideration of the individual's *experience*. Clinical textbooks tend to rely on describing the form of such experiences in mental health rather than the content (Crawford and Baker, 2009; Tischler, 2010, p. 3). As Oyebode suggests: 'What the arts and humanities can do for psychiatry is to reinforce the importance of the subjective' (2009, p. viii) – this is of course vital across all health-care encounters. One person's journey to diagnosis, through illness, and either into recovery, remission or readjustment to long-term challenges, will always be different to the next person's, even if their diagnosis, blood test or scan results are identical. Of course, it would be a poor clinician indeed who assumed that all people diagnosed with, for example, bowel cancer experience it identically. Yet despite the seeming obviousness of this fact, we often find our students undertaking clinical professional qualifications (mental health nursing – PC and CB – but also those in medicine and psychology – VT and BB) generally prefer – or even rely more on – the 'objective' reporting of medical notes, handover reports, and textbook formulations: that is, what they perceive as 'knowledge' about certain disorders, with the person's account or experience seen as perhaps important but *secondary*, and a fictional account even further distanced in relevance to their clinical practice. They sometimes *doubt* the subjective accounts, feeling that if someone is unwell with a mental health issue or confused as a result of a physical condition or anaesthesia, then their version may be skewed, their perceptions somewhat untrustworthy. Literature can promote and act as a reminder of the important, but often overlooked, idea that listening to, hearing, and valuing someone's own experience *even if it is not the 'objective' truth of the event* is not only crucial to developing a therapeutic relationship, but the most important element of the multiple narratives that develop and involve individuals who encounter various professionals. Privileging individuals' own recounting, formulation, interpretation and depiction of the life around the 'illness' is the foundation of narrative-based medicine – it can also be the foundation of narrative nursing and healthcare (Charon, 2006b; Hamkins, 2014; Kleinman, 1998).

A second core function is the enablement and promotion of reflection through narratives on a student's own values, life experience, expectations, assumptions and knowledge basis. Reflective capacity is a vital element not only of effective practice but also of building self-awareness, self-efficacy and resilience (Atkins and Murphy, 1993; Hannigan, 2001). Using literature to reflectively explore the subjective experiences of a range of people, attitudes, judgements witnessed in clinical placements, particular diagnoses, effective (and ineffective) reactions and responses that people have previously encountered, highlights the uniqueness and individuality of personal journeys. This in turn counterbalances the homogenising potential of symptomatological and diagnostic formulation. It may also act as a buffer to the current clinical stressors impacted upon by the austerity measures which risk effecting 'caring' to become secondary to 'cost saving' and 'efficiency' in under-staffed and stressful environments. Reflection through narratives also enables exploration of potentially challenging personal emotional responses and values through a safe medium. Reflecting on narratives invites, in turn, a storying of its own, a creative re-telling of personal and clinical experience. The teacher, supervisor or facilitator can subsequently, in hearing these creative reflective re-tellings, mirror the skills required to hear narrative accountings, and so the circularity of reflective practice and the promotion of narrative-based attending skills can continue.

An example of how literature can be used in clinical education and continuing professional development can be seen in the encounters professionals in almost all settings have with self-harm – that is, an injury or illness inflicted by a person on themselves for a range of different reasons, but not caused accidentally. It can be a challenging, stigmatised, anxiety-provoking experience to respond effectively to, and is one area in which narratives can be a particularly useful addition to aid students and professionals in reflecting on their own emotional reactions to the witnessing or finding of someone who has hurt themselves.

Teaching Mental Health Nursing Students about Self-Harm through Stories – CB's Experiences

Mental health nursing students often tell me that they hear some negative reactions towards people who self-harm – the act and, sometimes, the injury, becomes the focus of attention rather than the complex matrix of highly individual reasons, meaning and emotions experienced. They tell me that they hear staff suggesting that it is best *not* to ask the person about their self-harm, but are often unable to provide a rationale for this beyond the myth that self-harm is carried out 'for attention'. I use autobiographical narratives such as Caroline Kettlewell's *Skin Game* (1999) and Susanna Kaysen's *Girl, Interrupted* (1993), the collection I recently edited with many individuals with direct lived experience of self-harm (Baker et al., 2013) and fictional texts such as Rebecca Ray's *A Certain Age* (1998), to support students in considering some of the emotional and psychological wounds behind the visible; to think about how people come to a point where self-harm is the only viable way to cope with overwhelming emotions or traumatic experiences; and to consider how an approach which ignores the person behind the action may have profoundly dehumanising consequences. These stories – across a range of textual type – enable the students to not only consider their own values, but to interrogate some of the medical formulations of 'self-harm' (for example, the attribution of the label of 'personality disordered') in a critically reflective manner, remembering to prioritise not the *wound*, or the *diagnosis*, but the person, their distress, their strengths, their experiences and their often astonishing stories of survival and resilience. This in turn upends the predominant medical discourse they encounter and – hopefully – promotes a more empathic, critical and compassionate response in the future.

Narratives support the reflective exploration of different personal and professional responses to self-harm – the anxiety and fear around what may go wrong, the feeling of helplessness or frustration that someone is not 'feeling better' despite support, different professional reactions that are depicted as either helpful or unhelpful, or the 'what if you...' scenario which can in turn support empathic care.

Stories in Clinical Practice and Research

The foundation of healthcare practice, across all disciplines, should be based on hearing, respecting, valuing and responding to people's experiences, interpretations, relationships, priorities, emotions and life stories. Absorbing such emotive experiences necessitates a reflective capacity to enable effective responses, and developing this ability during clinical education is an important foundation for future critical, efficacious and reflective future practice (Atkins and Murphy, 1993; Hannigan, 2001). Hearing – not only *listening* for the particular details needed to formulate a care plan, assess risk or reach a diagnosis, but *hearing* the broader narrative – a person's own accounting of their illness and the life around it is a vital element of effective, ethical and humane healthcare generally (Charon, 2006b; Greenhalgh and Hurwitz, 1998; Kleinman, 1988b). This is the founding tenet of the well-established tradition of narrative medicine, whereby clinicians are encouraged not only to hold an interest in the life lived outside and around the medical condition, but to have degrees of narrative competence that enable them to effectively interpret, understand and reflect back people's experiences and their relationship to their illness (Frank, 1995). Charon suggests:

> Nonnarrative knowledge attempts to illuminate the universal by transcending the particular; narrative knowledge, by looking closely at individual human beings grappling with the conditions of life, attempts to illuminate the universals of the human condition by revealing the particular. (2006b, p. 9)

Hence, attention to the individual can tell us much about the collective. Charon argues that in medical and healthcare training, it is unrealistic to expect students to later contribute to necessary discussions around the complexities of service design, resource allocation and ethical treatments without first 'providing them with the skills of respecting multiple perspectives, hearing mediating competing voices, and recognizing and paying heed to a multitude of contradictory sources of authority' (2006b, p. 8). These are skills that can be developed through attention to narrative construction, portrayal and representation. The core features that literary scholars develop in applying and examining texts mirror those crucial for narrative-based practice – that is, attention to 'temporality, singularity, causality/contingency, intersubjectivity, and ethicality' (Charon, 2006b, p. 39). Drawing on the work of prominent literary theorist Jonathan Culler, Charon suggests that 'our "reading" of disease takes place at the level of the body's surface and its pathophysiological structure underneath the skin, while our reading of what a patient says takes place at the level of the evident meaning of the words and their implications buried in the clinical and/or personal state of affairs represented'; thus narrative medicine does not aim to teach future doctors to become literary theorists but instead to 'make them transparent to themselves as readers [...] we want to equip them with the skills to open up the stories of their patients to nuanced understandings and appreciation' (2006b, pp. 109–110). Charon's development of the 'parallel chart' demonstrates clearly how students' re-writing of the people they encounter, during which they learn to reflect not on the hospital record language of disease, neutrality and science, but the emotional reaction they have and consider the person to have instead, clearly shows these skills in action. That is, their focus on the unique, the subjective and the emotional and emotive subsequently can enable a longer-term focus on the individual *outside* of the tumour, the high blood pressure, anaemic blood panel or apparently strange belief system; a focus on the person, not the disease. More recently, work has been published on encouraging students to write their *own* pathography (Hwang et al., 2013). This study – which, interestingly, analysed the student's pathographies in terms of Hawkin's 1993 typography explored above, found that 'writing about an experience of illness allowed students to better understand patients' experience and to grow in self-understanding' (Hwang et al., 2013, p. 155).

Works on narrative medicine like Charon's predominantly focus on physical illness experience and more common psychological issues such as stress. This could be because mental health practitioners are seen as *necessarily* needing narrative competence – their entire practice is focused on listening to people and interpreting what they hear. But as Hamkins suggests, narrative psychiatry has benefits over the traditionally taught process of assessment, diagnosis and treatment. This does not, she explains, need to take the place of medication or of formal psychotherapies, but can instead form a connective and empowering therapeutic relationship where the focus begins with a person's strengths and tenacity, not their illness or 'deficits'. Hamkins not only demonstrates the practice of narrative psychiatry, but also circularly offers reflections from those people she works with, achieving mutuality in the therapeutic process. She writes: 'In narrative psychiatry, rather than privileging only stories of loss, suffering, conflict, neglect, or abuse in someone's life, I also search for stories of joy, connection, intimacy, consistency, and success, for these are the wealth of the people who consult with us. Instead of privileging a story of failure, we co-author a story of success in overcoming problems, no matter how small those successes may be' (Hamkins, 2014, p. 50). Like the focus on the individual who *has* the disease and how they experience, confront and live through or with it proposed by narrative medicine, in Hamkins' version of narrative psychiatry the entire focus is upended, from one of disorder, disease and disarray to one of strength, resourcefulness and survival. This acts as a promising new way of working in psychiatry and is adaptable across a range of different experiences and clinical disciplines. Of course, narrative *therapy* and the use of storytelling in therapy is more established as a psychotherapeutic practice (Crawford et al., 2004) – Hamkins differs in her focus of *all* psychiatric practice taking on these attentive and attending forms, aiding people to re-author their own stories and discover those stories of survival that they have, but which may be hidden under the self-consumptive nature of mental distress.

Paralleling the development of narrative healthcare is the use of narratives in health-based research, often in nursing care (Bold, 2012; Frid et al., 2000; Holloway and Freshwater, 2007a, 2007b; Overcash, 2004; Riessman, 2002; Sandelowski, 1991). This research draws upon literary strategies and readings to develop, inform or analyse the narratives of people experiencing illness, care, clinicians or hospital environments, facing death or experiencing long-term adjustments caused by illness or disease. This type of research does not aim to prove a hypothesis or to examine the efficacy of one treatment over another. In this respect, its apparent lack of 'scientific' rigour has meant that narrative research is relegated in the hierarchal family of evidence based practice to the status of a third cousin twice removed with the randomised controlled trial as the 'father'. This is evident, for example, in National Institute for Health and Clinical Excellence (NICE) guidelines which, for various reasons, can seem to tokenistically include the perspectives of people who use services, but then not to attend to their experiences in too much depth. Such research may focus on issues such as temporality, causality, individual experience, the emotional side of a diagnosis or disease, the role of the nurse or healthcare professional, or (more commonly perhaps) aim to draw together themes that naturalistically emerge from narratives of specific groups, for example women with breast cancer or young people who need to use genitourinary services (Holloway and Freshwater, 2007b). In nursing research, it is 'of concern', write Frid et al., 'to acknowledge the narrative's interpretative, temporal, action-oriented and ethical dimensions in the development of nursing knowledge' (2000, p. 701) – this valuing of the literary elements of the story contributes to a different kind of subjective knowledge-gathering that is important in planning and executing humane care. Holloway and Freshwater further this, suggesting value to the individual participant through the research process itself: through 'stories', 'participants in research come to understand their experience, legitimise their behaviour and share their emotional experience with others in holistic form which is not "fractured" or disrupted by researchers' (2007a, p. 703). And so the exploration of narrative and health comes full circle, returning to the personal and collective value of pathography.

Literature, Reading and Well-Being

It seems somewhat disingenuous to suggest that reading can be a healthy activity – as any book-lover will attest, reading is an activity that is relaxing, stimulating, educative, enjoyable and soothing (The Telegraph, 2009). Reading in a therapeutic sense is an area of only newly developing research, though in-depth studies are often either in development or published in non-traditional domains, leaving conclusions around the health benefits of reading somewhat tenuously drawn here, but strongly supported anecdotally. There is enormous scope here for applied practice within a health humanities ethos, in terms of the health and well-being benefits for people experiencing ill health, their informal carers, and those professionals allied to medicine such as care workers – all could benefit from the act of reading as in itself therapeutic and also as a tool for broadening empathy, knowledge and understanding, as suggested in depth above. Furthermore, there is potential for cost-effective but beneficial innovations in group reading activities, not only as already commonly exist in library settings through reading groups, but also those aimed at specific populations or those with similar shared experiences. The potential for increasing social integration and inclusion, shared communities of understanding, and mutual recovery through creative reading practice (where professionals and the people they support, as 'patients' and their carers, come together to benefit from each other's perspectives triggered through text) is enormous. The evidence is currently lacking – the opportunities are vast.

There is a broad evidence base for the health and well-being benefits and effectiveness of bibliotherapy and self-help cognitive behavioural therapy (Floyd, 2003; Frieswijk et al., 2006; Jamison and Scogin, 1995; Williams, 2001). Similarly, in the UK, Books on Prescription (BOP) schemes are now a feature of all libraries in England and Wales (Hicks, 2006; Hicks et al., 2010). Developed by Professor Neil Frude, BOP involves a general practitioner or other health professional prescribing a cognitive behavioural therapy self-help book from an expertly developed list as adjunctive or alternative treatment for mild to moderate mental health issues such as mild anxiety or depression – this is then collected from the person's local library (Frude, 2004). The 2004 NICE guidelines for the management of anxiety and related disorders (NICE, 2004) recommend this type of bibliotherapy for mild to moderate mental illness, and evidence suggests that BOP schemes are worthwhile and beneficial (Chamberlain et al., 2008).

Research carried out by Hicks and others suggests that the library is also a space where such work can more effectively occur as it is a neutral community space (Hicks et al., 2010), which may also improve social inclusion and support the development of social relationships (Anton, 2010). Arts interventions in libraries and similar public spaces have been shown to benefit older people (Aldridge and Dutton, 2009). Other forms of bibliotherapy such as reading group activities and the Mood Boosting Books (The Reading Agency, 2012) scheme are also commonly promoted in libraries (Hicks et al., 2010). The Mood Boosting Books scheme includes lists for young people and for carers too, marking an acknowledgement of the incredible challenges and rewards that being an informal carer can bring (see *A*'s experience in Chapter 8 – Case Study 8.1). Get Into Reading schemes have demonstrated that group reading of creative texts can have social and well-being benefits (Davis et al., 2008; Hodge et al., 2007). This model involves the reading out loud of texts, enabling those with low literacy levels to participate and invoking the memory of childhood story time, a soothing and incredibly beneficial activity for all children (Duursma et al., 2008).

Reading can act as a relaxing escape or as a form of self-directed therapy, alone or in groups, and further research into this field is very much warranted to examine a range of areas – in part to then subsequently convince policymakers and funders that reading is both important and cost saving. The reading process itself would be useful to examine – is it the type of reading material or the act of reading that provides relaxation; what well-being benefits are there in areas such as mood, anxiety, blood pressure and heart rate? Does reading in groups provide increased social capital and well-being over and above those attained through solo reading activity? Would reading groups in inpatient and outpatient settings improve the experiences of those using, for example, mental health services, attending chronic pain clinics or receiving chemotherapy? Is there an element of *mutual recovery* possible through the shared reading experience of professionals and the people they care for – and how does the reciprocality of this arrangement deconstruct traditional hierarchies of care? A wealth of possibilities are available here with great potential to evidence base the therapeutic and well-being effects of reading.

Summary and Conclusions

The successful continuance, since its launch in 1982, of the US-based journal *Literature and Medicine* – and the range of literary-focused papers in both the *Journal of Medical Humanities* and *Medical Humanities* – attests to the enduring scholarly interest in the literary portrayal of illness, health, death, disability and survival. As Charon suggests, 'The field's impressive growth in the past 25 years attests to the urgency and timeliness of literature's contributions to medicine, a contribution that can provide medical students and doctors with the narrative skills necessary for effective medicine and with stories resonant with the human meanings of illness' (2000, p. 23). Like the literary interest in feminism, colonialism, diversity, language, interrelationships, love, sex and death, pathographism is a literary phenomenon and genre demonstrated as worthy of its own branch of study. Such interest does not reside solely in the realm of literary and academic interpretation of specific canonical texts or collections of material, or in the value of the sense-making act of writing one's own pathography. As demonstrated in this chapter, in the past 20 years or so there has been an increasing focus on the value of narrative, literature and narrative competence for and in clinical education and practice – on what literature can tell us about human experiences that test the limits of strength and endurance, survival and defeat, and how literature can support, develop and promote humane, empathic and reflective capacities for clinicians and students. As the focus of medicine moves from viewing the *patient* as a body, a constellation of symptoms, a syndrome or a diagnosis, towards seeing the *person* as an autonomous and active partner in their care, literature can tell us much about the lived experience of that person *outside* and *beyond* the biomedical gaze. Reminding us of the value of compassion, holism, listening and hearing, individualism, of the chaos that sickness brings into the lived life through its interruption to health, literature is a valuable tool for self-reflection and potentially provides a box of skills and materials for use in the therapeutic relationship. Of course, therapeutic relationships work in many different ways – from the student in the day surgery unit who cares for a new person daily, the GP who has 10 minutes per person, to the psychotherapist who spends several years supporting an individual – but all can use literature in a range of ways. Both storytelling and the reading of resultant literary forms are a salve for the most wounded of souls, the wounded healer, the wounded carer, the observer interested in wounds. Stories will never cease to be told – unique as they are – as people continue to experience birth, life, sickness and death.

4
Narrative and Applied Linguistics

In Chapter 3 we saw how narratives in fiction and in biographical writing have a role to play in the health humanities. In this chapter we will pursue the question of narrative a little further and consider the role it plays in shaping and helping us interpret the experience of illness, and the value of a narrative approach in helping us create a genuinely humanitarian healthcare.

Whilst narrative medicine and the narrative turn has taken hold in healthcare research and practice in the last couple of decades, it has of course had a much longer pedigree. The 1980s and 1990s saw a narrative renaissance in medicine, nursing and related disciplines such as occupational therapy, psychotherapy and even physiotherapy. Yet this was a re-birth rather than a process of starting from scratch. In the late 20th-century narrative turn there were echoes of movement which had started a century earlier. In 1869, Armand Trousseau, the French internist described as 'the leader of the French therapeutic Renaissance' (Karkabi and Castel, 2013, p. 356), wrote a textbook on clinical medicine and therapeutics in which he insisted on linking science and the arts in medicine. He said: '...every science touches art at some points. Every art has its scientific side; the worst man of science is he who is never an artist, and the worst artist is he who is never a man of science' (1869, p. 40). Similarly the physician William Osler, in a lecture given in his capacity as the President of the British Classical Association, said: 'Now, the men in your guild secrete materials which do for society at large what the thyroid gland does for the individual. The humanities are the hormones' (1920, p. 26). Osler, who was believed to have originated the phrase 'listen to your patient: he is telling you the diagnosis', was a passionate believer in the educational and diagnostic value of patients' accounts, and was also a believer in the value of the arts and humanities in medicine, and the role of the arts in deepening compassion and empathy. These aspects of the healing arts in healthcare were given a boost in the late 20th century by Rita Charon, who we met in Chapter 3. As she put it:

> Along with scientific ability, physicians need the ability to listen to the narratives of the patient, grasp and honour their meanings, and be moved to act on the patient's behalf. This is narrative competence, that is, the competence that human beings use to absorb, interpret, and respond to stories. [...] it enables the physician to practice medicine with empathy, reflection, professionalism, and trustworthiness. Such a medicine can be called *narrative medicine*. (Charon, 2001, p. 1897)

Put crudely, narratives are the stories that people tell about their lives (Gray et al., 2005); or as Prince put it, 'The recounting ... of one or more real or fictitious events...' (Prince, 1991, p. 58). Some would argue this definition is incomplete and that a text should describe at least two events for it to be considered a narrative (Barthes, 1982; Rimmon-Kenan, 2002). Frid et al. (2000) add the importance of a point of view, and that this is what distinguishes narratives from stories: 'narrative is an account of events experienced by the narrator', while storytelling is 'the repeated telling or reading of a story by persons other than the narrator' (p. 695). Paley and Eva (2005, p. 86) add more:

> What is required, we think, is the sense of one thing leading to another; the idea that something happened as a result of something else (which is absent from the nurse/doctor example above). In saying this, we are agreeing with another group of critics who argue, not only that a narrative must include reference to two or more events, but also that some of those events must be causally related (Bal, 1985; Richardson, 1997).

Barbara Herrnstein Smith (1981, p. 228) defines narrative discourse as 'someone telling someone else that something happened', emphasising how narrative involves a teller and a listener, a writer and a reader in some sort of communicative relationship.

Veteran qualitative researcher Norman Denzin (1989, p. 37) provides the following definition:

> A 'narrative' is a story that tells a sequence of events that are significant for the narrator and his or her audience. A narrative as a story has a plot, a beginning, a middle and an end. It has an internal logic that makes sense to the narrator. A narrative relates events in a temporal, causal sequence. Every narrative describes a sequence of events that have happened.

In the study of healthcare, narrative theory has been deployed extensively over the last couple of decades to understand the first-hand experience of illness (McLeod, 2000). This has been accompanied by an increasing belief that narratives are an important means by which we make our existence intelligible and meaningful (Polkinghorne, 1988). 'The narrative provides meaning, context, and perspective for the patient's predicament' (Greenhalgh and Hurwitz, 1999, p. 48). Earlier work sought to create the basis of a narrative approach and theory in the social sciences as an alternative to the then dominant positivistic approach (Sarbin, 1986). One of the key individuals in the development of the narrative approach in the social sciences was Jerome Bruner, who had previously had a distinguished career as a cognitive scientist. In his later career he became interested in the idea of narrative and argued for its role as an alternative to the predominant scientific understanding of the world (Bruner, 1990). Seeing the human world in terms of the stories people tell means that the analyst is attentive to the way these tend to have a beginning, a middle and an end (Riessman, 1993). The narrative approach also encourages us to consider how the various stories told by people have common elements or episodes – a core story, comprising the main points the teller is conveying. Labov and Waletzky (1967) claimed that the key elements of a story are: abstract, orientation, complicating action, resolution, evaluation and coda. In his classic analysis of folk tales Vladimir Propp (1968) identified 31 elements in a folktale, including such aspects as the hero leaving home on an adventure, being thwarted or injured by a villain, acquiring a magical device or assistant to help him in his quest, successfully overcoming the villain and getting married at the end. These kinds of approaches tend to focus on form and structure, language and grammar and have been criticised for detracting from the function and importance of the narrative itself (Priest et al., 2002).

The Devil is in the Detail: Making Sense of Health and Illness Experiences

Whilst the early days of interest in narratives in healthcare were full of brave manifestos for the value of the approach, the 21st century has seen a focus on the narratives associated with specific groups of people with particular conditions. For example, Hinder and Greenhalgh (2012) looked at the tales told by people with diabetes and other health and social problems. On examining how people talked about their diabetes in the context of their often difficult lives, Hinder and Greenhalgh were able to identify some common features of the experience, or at least the way the tale was told to the researchers:

> Many participants talked of 'balance'. But in contrast to the bio-medical meaning of this term (physiological homeostasis), they saw self-management as relating to balance in their wider lives, including controlling personal stress levels, nurturing family and social relationships and achieving work–life balance. One aspect of 'balance', for example, was between the immediate physical pleasure and social significance of food treats and the deferred benefits of a strict dietary regimen. (Hinder and Greenhalgh, 2012, p. 8)

Thus, inspired by the narrative approach, the researchers have been able to identify common features in the way that participants tell the stories of their present-day lives. Managing family relationships, looking after oneself and having treats as well as managing the diabetes were sometimes in tension and the participants juggled these with varying levels of success. The experience of having conditions like these does not necessarily yield the kind of narrative that has a happy ending like the traditional folktale.

Another example of how an attention to narratives in healthcare can yield unexpected insights comes from Rich and Grey (2003), who provide a fascinating account of the life-worlds of young men in the United States who had been subject to what they called 'penetrating violence', namely stabbings and gunshot wounds. Whilst there is a great deal of research, practice and technique to deal with the bodily aspects of these injuries, we know far less about what it means from the point of view of the sufferers. Moreover, given the socioeconomic and ethnic divisions in the US, many of these young men had little or no first-hand exposure to healthcare in any form prior to the incident, nor had they acquired informal health knowledge from friends or family members. People in socioeconomically disadvantaged positions in the US often have very limited access indeed to healthcare. Whereas this patient group is often seen to be difficult, being challenging and noncompliant, and at risk of recurrent injury if the wounds occur as part of an ongoing dispute, their experiences in hospital may affect them profoundly. Earl, a 23-year-old man who was stabbed while walking to a local store, described the incident as follows:

> So I didn't really think I was facing death, y'know?
> Till when, after I was waitin' for the ambulance to come,
> I started gettin' really, really cold?
> And I felt like I was goin' to faint.
> And the officer was talkin' to me,
> and as I was goin' down on my knees,
> I heard him sayin', "Oh, he's not gonna make it.
> He's not gonna make it."
> And that's when I got scared. (Rich and Grey, 2003, p. 959)

Whilst some young men who survive such assaults have been said by health professionals to wear their scars as badges of honour and talk as if they were invulnerable, at the time they are injured they often express fear about the possibility of death which may set in well before the ambulance arrives or the hospital procedures commence. Whilst they may later express a degree of bravado about their ordeal, at the time they may be very vulnerable and appreciate the human touch of particular healthcare personnel:

> The doctor was good.
> Who's the doctor with the glasses?
> Well, when I got to the hospital,

he made me feel a lot better here
'Cause he was holdin' my hand,
he kept tellin' me, "just hold on.
You're gonna be alright.
I ain't gonna let you die."
He just kept tellin' me,
kept tellin' me that.
That made me feel a lot better.
A lot better. (Rich and Grey, 2003, p. 960)

Rich and Grey say that not only is this kind of thing reassuring in its own right, but it also made the patient better able to cope with the invasive and complex procedures he had to undergo in hospital later. The role that healthcare providers can play during the 'window of vulnerability' that opens during the days and weeks after injury represents an important opportunity for further narrative investigation (Rich and Grey, 2003, p. 960). It may for example offer further insight into how the experience of life-threatening injury is assimilated into the person's life story and how the likelihood of ongoing conflict with other young men and consequent re-victimisation may be averted.

Narrating Life-Threatening Illness: Cancer Narratives

There are some kinds of problems and conditions that have been especially well studied by means of narrative. Cancer has been subject to a variety of investigations from a narrative point of view. Indeed, it is as if cancer, and cancer narratives, represent the ideal type of narrative study of illness, from which other types derive. We will write later about some other kinds of problems that have been far less well studied, but for the moment let us examine how cancer experiences have yielded developments in the study of illness narratives. One of the classic works in this area was Arthur Frank's *The Wounded Storyteller* (Frank, 1995). Here, as we described in Chapter 3, Frank describes three different kinds of narrative that may be found when people describe their illness experience: the restitution narrative, the chaos narrative and the quest narrative.

Frank's (1995) 'restitution narrative' of illness is one in which a previously healthy person becomes ill, is diagnosed, treated and restored to health. In a similar way to that in which the sick role includes a suite of rights and duties governing how sick individuals are expected and allowed to behave, being healthy and a 'survivor' also places moral expectations on the person (Frank, 2003). For example, Kaiser (2008) points to the frequent images in the popular media of cancer 'survivors' as being happy and heroic, participating in sporting events that demonstrate exceptional health and fitness in the face of illness. These kinds of images, and the dominant frame of survivorship in which cancer is 'beaten' or 'conquered', tend to support the medical model of disease and the capability of medicine to triumph over cancer and restore health (Kaiser, 2008). These phenomena represent a particularly widely disseminated example of the 'restitution narrative'.

In the chaos narrative, by contrast, the key feature is that life will not get better and that no one is in control, least of all the patient. In this kind of narrative sufferers describe an 'emotional battering' (Frank, 1995, p. 101). This may come about through the way that health professionals appear to be rejecting or failing to understand their suffering or from their social exclusion by others. In the chaos narrative, the sufferer may attempt to reintroduce predictability but this is not usually possible, and these efforts have a cost for the individual. Chaos narratives disclose vulnerability, futility and ineffectiveness (Frank, 1995, p. 97) and can be difficult to listen to. In contrast to restitution narratives which describe illness as transitory, they depict people as if they had been 'sucked into the undertow of illness' (Frank, 1995, p. 115).

For example, in a study of cancer sufferers by Brown and De Graaf (2013) one of their participants said:

> *Sanne*: You always hope that you can have a bit longer [participant becomes emotional at this point]. See, I know well that if you enter into chemo and you're getting better, then you know why you're doing chemo. But what if you're not getting better? Of course that is really hard. You just hope that you can have a bit longer. Yeah, then, it is important that, see, you never really know how it is going ... an oncologist doesn't really know, no one really knows... The family doctor doesn't know. All of us, we just don't know! (Brown and De Graaf, 2013, p. 550)

Here, there is an emphasis on not knowing, on the part both of the oncologist and of himself, the fact that chemotherapy is apparently not leading to progress and the difficulty of sustaining hope. This then could be seen as an example of what Frank might call 'chaos' – there is no orderly progress towards restitution or changed identity.

The third type of narrative described by Frank is what he calls the 'quest narrative', which describes the situation where the individual accepts illness, and tries to use this, in the belief that something can be gained through the illness experience. Thus, illness is understood as a challenge and an opportunity for change (Frank, 1995, p. 166). The difference between this and the restitution narrative is that sufferers are not seeking recovery as a sole end point. Frank proposes three variants of the quest narrative. The first is the memoir in which events are simply related. Second, there is the manifesto in which illness is understood to be a cue for social action or change. Thirdly there is the automythology in which illness is formulated as revealing fate or destiny (Frank, 1995, pp. 119–120). In the quest narrative, the person whilst no longer ill retains the marks of illness – rather like how in other storytelling traditions a hero's status depends on his having been initiated through agony to atonement. We might see this kind of story in the commonly used phrase 'having cancer is the best thing that happened to me' and its usual accompaniment of how illness encouraged the sufferer to reorient their life, do something different or reappraise their values. When this is the primary narrative put forward by the sufferer Frank would encourage us to be sceptical. This, says Frank, demands critical evaluation as to how the move has been accomplished straight from the onset of symptoms to a quest narrative without apparent suffering – this, he says, appears 'too clean cut' (Frank, 1995, p. 135).

Of course, Frank's different sorts of illness narratives are ideal types, and any real life story of how a person's illness has progressed may well involve elements of a number of these idealisations. Moreover they do not cover all detailed aspects of the story of an episode of illness such as cancer. Even when the prospects of survival are bleak and there is not the kind of resolution found in the restitution or quest narratives, there still may be a sense of order and meaning. Ho et al. (2013) report a study of Chinese patients with terminal cancer, many of whom were living in nursing homes with limited comforts, yet who managed to find meaning in their situation even though the limited prospects and terminal nature of their condition might lend themselves to a 'chaos narrative' in Frank's typology. Often it was simple things like family life that were identified as being especially important. As one 82-year-old man said:

> The happiest times in my life now are when my youngest daughter comes and visits. I didn't spend a lot of time with her when she was young as I used to travel a lot in my work. We barely had any time to talk or see each other back then... I hope that she understands me and that I am a good father who cares deeply about her. (Ho et al., 2013, p. 962)

Thus it is not inevitable that an apparently hopeless situation yields a hopeless narrative. It is through these ongoing stories of family life and continuing contact with relatives that, as Ho et al. put it, people are enabled to live through this liminal stage of the end of life with a sense of dignity and meaning.

In common with attempts to grapple with narrative medicine in the 1990s, Frank (1995) is, in a sense, trying to address the big picture and characterise the shape and form of illness narratives as a whole. By contrast, many contemporary accounts of cancer narratives tend to focus not on describing this big picture, but instead on characterising aspects of the patient journey in more detail. To take an example of this, let us consider a paper by Sinding (2014) about cancer experience which focused on what patients wanted from their healthcare providers. One of the major dilemmas the participants faced concerned the role of choice in the care they were receiving and the degree of responsibility they felt was being pressed upon them. In recent years healthcare providers have placed a good deal of emphasis on informed consent in such cases, where patients are informed of the risks and benefits of different courses of action but are encouraged to make their own decisions. In some healthcare jurisdictions there is a growing sense that patients are having to act as their own care managers as they navigate through a complex mosaic of statutory, private and charitable provision. Sinding (2014) was working in Canada, where one support organisation for sufferers says:

> The Canadian cancer care system is increasingly complex. Often, there is no single 'case manager' or 'patient advocate' to help

you to manage your care from diagnosis through treatment and beyond. As a result, you may find that you must advocate for yourself and take an active role in the coordination of your care... Self-advocacy means taking an active role in your treatment to make sure you get the support and care you need. (Willow Breast Cancer Support, 2010, p. 5)

Whereas patients appreciated the value of choice at one level, there was a sense from many of Sinding's participants that they would also have appreciated more guidance through the process, and sometimes felt that healthcare providers were leaving them to puzzle things out on their own:

And then he said, 'and I'm not saying any more, that's all, here's your task you go off and think about that.' Which I actually thought was pretty good. The only problem was he didn't say, 'and this is where you should look for some of those answers.' And yet he is very, I mean you hear about surgeons not being empathetic and I think he's got quite a lot of empathy but just, you know and he has pamphlets outside in the office, you know breast cancer support services, so he has all this stuff, but it would have been... Now he did say, 'you should go talk to people.' He did say you know 'call me any time.' So he did, but you know at that point you're saying: yea but, like can you just like give me a phone number or walk me [there]? (Sinding, 2014, pp. 64–65)

This was a theme that cropped up in a number of patients' narratives. They felt that they would have liked healthcare providers to 'walk with' or 'walk alongside' them a little more. Moreover, whilst they felt they had been given choice they found themselves wanting more guidance from the health professionals about what the best option might be – in other words what the doctor him or herself would 'vote' for. Accordingly, as a result of attention to these patients' narratives, Sinding (2014) attempts to reformulate the relationship between autonomy, informed consent and paternalism in healthcare. Whilst contemporary healthcare providers are understandably reluctant to force particular treatment options on patients and there is a good deal of emphasis on autonomy, it is equally an ethical concern that patients should not feel abandoned. Patients seemed to want professionals – not just doctors and nurses but receptionists, technicians and other ancillary staff – to have a greater appreciation of the state of mind they would be in, and pay attention to the patient and not to the computer screen. Sinding's approach draws attention to the vulnerability that often accompanies life-threatening illness and the complexity and uncertainty associated with many decisions. Perhaps, she suggests, more empathy, compassion and involvement on the part of staff, rather than enhancing paternalism, might even promote the value of genuine patient autonomy.

The predominant narratives of cancer experience do not suit everyone. Narrative can be about difference, division and exclusion as well. The predominant narratives of a condition like cancer – fighting it, beating it and running marathons, changing one's priorities and lifestyle and coming out cleansed – do not suit everyone's experience. A variety of dimensions such as gender, race and socioeconomic position can intersect to make particular people's experiences unique and at odds with the predominant way in which their situation is understood. In her memoir *The Cancer Journals*, Audre Lorde (1980, p. 25) asserted that every part of her identity as 'black feminist mother lover poet' must be accommodated in understanding her breast cancer experience. The organisations through which treatment was administered for Lorde's illness did not occupy the same social position or ideological perspective as their patient. Lorde felt marginalised in a system that prioritised beauty over health, heterosexual concerns over lesbian needs, and white women's circumstances over those of black women. Consequently, as well as being an account of her journey as a patient, Lorde's book is a manifesto for institutional change. It is also a testament to the ways in which the multi-layered identity she ascribed to herself constructs her path through illness.

Hidden Suffering, Hidden Stoicism: Narratives of Healthcare-Associated Infections

Cancer has been the subject of a great deal of study such that any literature search with terms like 'cancer', experience' and 'narrative' yields a large number of items. Yet there are other areas which have been neglected in the rush to capture the patient narrative. The experience of iatrogenic problems has not been so widely explored. In particular infections acquired whilst in hospital have not been subject to a very high level of scrutiny from the patients' point of view. When the present authors began to explore this in detail a couple of years ago there was very little in the literature. The few studies in existence suggested that patients were apt to highlight their desire for information and communication from healthcare personnel (Burnett et al., 2010; Skyman et al., 2010) yet this is not always forthcoming (Gardner and Cook, 2004). Patients with healthcare-associated infections (HCAIs) have also reported a sense of violation or betrayal at having contracted an infection while in hospital (Skyman et al., 2010). In Andersson et al.'s (2011) study, participants identified what they saw to be a lack of knowledge on the part of staff where HCAIs were concerned and the staff were blamed for inconsistent and ineffective hygiene procedures. In Skyman et al.'s (2010) work, patients were additionally put out by the cancellation or postponement of the treatment for their original complaint as a result of their infection. As might be expected, patients suffering an infection reported more depressive and anxious symptoms than those without (Tarzi et al., 2001) as well as a loss of confidence in the health service where HCAIs are concerned, and their dread of going back to hospital (Burnett et al., 2010).

Accordingly we (Brown et al., in press) conducted exploratory interviews with people who had suffered surgical site infections. What was notable from the outset was that the participants exhibited a great deal of stoicism. Rather than saying the hospital or healthcare personnel were at fault, they were much more likely to attribute the infection to chance:

> *Interviewer:* Why do you think you got an infection?
> *Participant 1:* I don't know. It was just one of those things. I think it happened when I was in the operating theatre because the surgeon said 'you've broken my record, you're my first patient to get one of these'. The doctors and nurses were very good, they were very concerned. I don't think it was the surgeon's fault. I think it was just something that happens, during the operation, it's just germs flying around and they picked me.

In tandem with this tendency to attribute a surgical site infection to 'just something that happens' was a tendency to accept the suffering involved with a high degree of stoicism and equanimity. One participant had undergone abdominal surgery to deal with a tumour and the wound would not stay closed due to infection. Despite suspicions that this had resulted from poor surgical wound closure techniques, he had decided against complaint:

> Our eldest daughter who was a nurse for 30 years said I should write a letter of complaint but I don't feel like sitting down writing it. And where is it going to get me? The surgeon I understand is about the top man in the infirmary so he ought to know what he is doing. (Brown et al., in press)

Complaint then is formulated as being ineffective, especially in the face of the expertise of the medical profession. This tendency to attribute surgical site infection to bad luck and to avoid getting angry with the hospital meant that participants and their families were absorbing a great deal of pain and incapacity themselves in such a way as not to trouble the hospital. In other words, attention to the patients' narratives yielded a good deal of insight as to how the pain and disability associated with HCAIs was being accommodated in the context of their lives and their dealings with the hospital.

The contemporary trend towards examining, exploring and showcasing patients' narratives in healthcare has often been seen as empowering for patients. Returning for a moment to Rita Charon's work, she put it this way:

> Certainly, more and more patients have insisted on achieving a narrative mastery over the events of illness, not only to unburden themselves of painful thoughts and feelings but, more fundamentally, to claim such events as parts, however unwelcome, of their lives. (Charon, 2001, p. 1901)

Narrative approaches with an emphasis on preserving rather than dismembering the stories that are told, as Gray et al. (2005, p. 73) suggest, make the study of healthcare 'more relevant to the actual lives of ill people'. Moreover, it addresses factors which are of socio-political significance too. It is through language that power relationships are acted out: 'linguistic exchanges are also relations of symbolic power in which the power relations between speakers or their respective groups are actualised' (Bourdieu, 1991, p. 37).

Co-Construction and Co-Production: Narrative as a Joint Enterprise

So far we have been considering narratives and stories as if they were produced by patients more or less spontaneously. However, in practice, healthcare consultations are considerably more complex than this and the picture is built up as a result of an intimate interactive dance where questions and responses combine to produce a joint synthesis of what the problem is, what the consultation is about, and what the course of action should be.

Consequently a more detailed sociolinguistic approach has been favoured by many authors who are seeking to characterise the 'grain' of conversation in healthcare encounters between patients and different professional groups. Whereas it is very often doctors whose work with patients has been studied in this way, some authors are studying nurses and other professional groups too. An example of this can be found in the work of Collins (2005), who provides instances of encounters between professionals and clients in diabetes care. In one example Collins draws the reader's attention to the differences between an encounter involving a nurse and one involving a doctor. Collins notes that several distinctions are apparent between the nurse's and the doctor's communications and their respective forms of explanation. In each excerpt, the patient is positioned differently in the construction of the assessment and accompanying explanations. In the nurse consultation, the patient is invited to contribute and presents the contrast between two possible formulations (I thought I'd done alright, but you say I haven't), and his interpretation helps manoeuvre the nurse's explanation into position, so that it represents a response that reconciles these apparently contrasting patient and professional viewpoints. By contrast, the doctor's explanations are not developed from the patient's talk but instead the patient's assessment follows the doctor's, so he confirms rather than redresses or expands the assessment and explanations the doctor provides. In summary then, Collins (2005) argues that the nurse's consultation proceeds with the patient's responsibility and behaviour whilst the doctor's consultation is dominated by biomedical assessments and interventions. This is reflected by the different linguistic constructions that each professional uses: the doctor deploys a more technical and specialised language, while the nurse employs language more redolent of everyday usage. She uses some of the same words the patient has employed in the surrounding talk. This joint construction of health and illness stories is not confined to interactions between health professionals and clients. As Dew et al. (2014) note, there is a good deal of interaction about health and illness issues that goes on among family members, work colleagues and other acquaintances which helps to set the tone, frame the explanations and discern possible remedies and courses of action. As one participant said:

> [...] at work you'll be sitting at the table and you'll find out this person has done this or found out that and I'll always ask... 'How did you find it? Have you used it for long?' and I just put that in my memory bank. (Dew et al., 2014, p. 37)

Thus, narratives are assembled in a variety of ways, with resources culled from family members, friends, work colleagues and the wider culture. As Dew et al. (2014) report, these kinds of accounts are a kind of mosaic or 'hybrid', incorporating both folk and medical knowledge which participants collectively have at their disposal for addressing health problems.

Linguistic Techniques and New Evidence: A Corpus Approach to Adolescent Health

Discussions about health, healthcare problems and pleas for help are not necessarily organised into a story of the kind which is easily susceptible to narrative analysis. Nevertheless, an attention to language form and content can be invaluable to healthcare researchers and practitioners seeking to understand health. To illustrate different dimensions of the analysis of language, let us take an example once again from our own work applying a technique from language study and second language learning to the exploration of healthcare language. The approach we have used is one where a large body or corpus of language is systematically explored for the insight it can give about how a language is used, how terms are deployed, what forms and words tend to occur together, the concepts into which the language can be formulated and so on. Publishers of dictionaries have been aware of the value of this for some time in learning about what words are used and what they mean in a particular language community, and it has been gaining ground in second language learning and teaching. Over the last few years we have been applying this technique to the analysis of healthcare language. We have collaborated with the proprietors of a website set up to offer health advice to young people, www.teenage healthfreak.org.uk, which, among various other features, offers an online agony aunt service. Over the period 2004 to 2008 we were able to interrogate a 1.6 million word corpus of questions written in to the website by its users. The data therefore provide a substantial snapshot of contemporary health concerns communicated on a regular basis by the teenage contributors. The examples and analysis we will consider here come from Harvey and Brown (2012).

To begin interrogating this substantial body of language, we generated a list of keywords which provide a thematic characterisation of the language. Keywords, according to McCarthy and Handford, are words which 'best define' (2004, p. 174) a text or texts – words that are significantly higher in one language data set compared with another. Keywords are an important indicator of both expression and content (Seale et al., 2007) and have been used by an increasing number of researchers as a reliable means of identifying key themes in characterising health language corpora (Adolphs et al., 2004; Harvey et al., 2007; Seale, 2006; Seale et al., 2007). In this sense, a 'keyword' is one which is statistically more frequent, rather than the usual sense of words deemed to be of significant social and cultural importance. Table 4.1 presents a representative overview of these keywords resolved into health-related themes.

As can be seen from Table 4.1, the most frequently occurring terms can be grouped into meaningful clusters of content items indicative of the central health issues which concern the website users. Although informed by clearly defined semantic areas, the categories overlap to some extent. For example, mental health, body image, drugs and alcohol all have links to mental health. Clearly, reproductive health yielded a great many queries. We have discussed these at greater length elsewhere (Harvey et al., 2007). Here, let us follow Harvey and Brown (2012) and consider what the Teenage Health Freak corpus can tell us about self-injury. Given the prevalence of the phenomenon in the contemporary era it is not surprising that in a corpus of this size there were examples of people describing and soliciting help for their self-injury. In Box 4.1 we

Table 4.1 Keywords by categorisation of health themes in adolescent health emails

Theme	Examples of keywords
Sexual health	Sex, sexual, penis, pregnant, period, orgasm, AIDS, infertile, STD, STI, sperm, contraception, HIV, clitoris, vagina, vulva, PMS, erection, condom, masturbate, gay, abortion, foreplay, intercourse, virgin, unprotected, lesbian, oral, pill, ovulation, herpes, thrush, chlamydia, pregnancy, tampon, testicles, genitalia, viagra, scrotum, labia, glans, ovaries, foreskin, balls, fanny, bisexual, miscarriage
Mental health	Depression, depressed, suicide, suicidal, die, overdose, antidepressants, cut, cuts, cutting, self-harm, scars, prozac, sad, unhappy, self, harm, wrists, addiction, addict, stress, stressed, ADHD, paranoid, mental, mad, moods, sad, unhappy, crying, personality, anxiety
Body weight/image	Anorexia, anorexic, weight, size, overweight, fat, obese, underweight, skinny, thin, bulimia, BMI, exercise, diets, kilograms, KG, KGS, bulimia, calories
Drugs/alcohol	Drugs, cannabis, cocaine, heroin, pills, alcohol, drunk, drinking, poppers, mushrooms, marijuana, crack, ecstasy, addict, stoned, LSD, cigarettes, dope
Serious conditions	Cancer, epilepsy, diabetes, anthrax
Minor conditions	Acne, zits, blackhead, mumps, scabies, dandruff, worms, cystitis
Medication	Medicine, medication, prescribed, antibiotics, tablets, pill, pills

Source: Harvey and Brown (2012, p. 322).

present some data from Harvey and Brown (2012) where we have examined the occurrence of self-harm with terms such as 'help' and 'stop'. We selected these terms because they appeared to offer some potential for insight into the dilemmas surrounding the desire to give up self-harm and adopt different coping mechanisms that do not involve self-injury.

The examples in Box 4.1 provide more detail concerning personal experiences of self-harm, with several persistent new themes emerging. For example, self-harm is presented as a response to physical and sexual abuse, verbal bullying, family turmoil, as well as being a reaction to feeling upset and depressed. Self-harm is constructed as a survival mechanism, a form of relief, or as one of the contributors above

Box 4.1 Examples of messages containing the common collocates 'help' and 'stop'

- i tried to **stop self harming**, and i managed 5 weeks 3 days, and i failed after that, and i know ive let myself down but alot has happened to me, which made me self harm in the first place, i kept things inside me for soo long, and i have suport from skool which is gr8 help, like i have my mentor and another teacher, but recently ive started to keep it inside me and is making me self harm, and i always wrote to my teacher to say how i felt, but something stops me now, and the alternatives i used instead of **self harming** dont **help** nomore. what can i do. i know i need help, but i cant stay strong with the self harming, so much hurt is inside me and i cant get it out of my head. please please relpy!!
- i need 2 **cut** myself all the time. **help** me pls
- i have recently started **cutting** myself and i want to **stop** but i cant. ive treid loads of things and im woried becase when ever i get upset i start to visualise myslef cutting . and then when im alone if i havent calmed down i start **cutting** and i want to **stop**. i hate having to hide my **cuts**/scars and i need **help**
- i smoke but im not addicted it just makes me better as i get easily stressed. have you got any suggestions for things i could do instead because i started smoking to **stop** myself from **cutting** myself
- Doctor Ann: About a year ago I **stopd cutting** myself with a penknife because I'd managed to sort out my life. The other day my family had a row and I started to **cut** myself using kitchen knives, straight across my wrists. One of my friends saw the scars today, and everyone thinks I'm doing it for attention, but them thinking that partially lead to it anyway – it's a catch 22 situation **Help**!
- i got sexually abused when i was 5 till 11 and i cant get over it i've had coucnelling but it doesnt **help** now i just **cut** myself all the time to try and deal with it
- i get called names because i wear glasses and have ginger hair the name calling got so bad i have started to **cut** my wrists please **help**

- i keep going depressed. i get so upset now i start to heave, im on anti depressants but only been on them a week. i spent a year in hopsital to **help** with my **self-harming (cutting)** issues nothing has changed it has got worse and so has my ocd. just want to be happy and not so panicky and insecure
- CAN YOU **HELP** ME WITH **SELF HARMING** OR NOT ITS BEEN GOING ON KNOW FOR 3 YEARS AND I JUST CARNT STOP WHAT SHOULLD I DO CAN YOU HELP ME THANK YOU
- I've started slitting my wrists, it's my way of coping with my problems. But now I really want to stop the scars are really ugly!! But i duno how 2 i feel i need to **cut** or I'll break!!! Please **Help**!!!
- i self harm and i whant some **help** i hate my self for ding it it is like a vitiose circle is there any thing u can do that would help me to **stop** i do not whant to talk to my parents

Source: Harvey and Brown (2012, p. 326).

puts it, a means of trying 'to deal with it', in this instance, the trauma of sexual abuse. Self-harm also appears to serve as a visual manifestation of distress, although the actual physical injuries that speak for those who cut (Ross, 1994, p. 13) can also be a source of disquiet: 'I really want to stop the scars are really ugly!!', 'i hate having to hide my cuts/scars'. Thus these accounts reveal some of the intolerable circumstances of young people involved in self-harm. Although the act is portrayed as a survival mechanism, a response (no matter how 'maladaptive' to unbearable emotional distress (Favazza, 1996)), its legacy of cuts and scars, which have to be treated and hidden from others, only appears to aggravate the predicaments of these young people for whom self-harm is experienced as an effective form of relief. As one of the correspondents succinctly sums up their situation, 'it's a catch 22 situation Help!'

Interestingly, self-harm is also perceived to be an alternative to other risky behaviours. In an effort to avoid it, the adolescents seek participation in other deleterious activities, such as smoking. Yet, such is the pull of cutting, these substitutes are comparatively less compelling and so abandoned in favour of self-harming behaviours. As one of the adolescents comments: 'the alternatives i used instead of self harming dont help nomore' (sic). The pull of self-harm over and above these other risk behaviours can perhaps be further explained by the broad range of motives presented by the adolescents for the activity. As an antidote to psychological upheaval, self-harm is hard to replace since it can be caused for a number of reasons, while at the same time fulfilling different functions (Horne and Csipke, 2009, p. 656), be it emotional release or articulating (such as visualising) inexpressible distress.

Data sets such as we have described here from Harvey and Brown (2012) can have a valuable contribution to make to the education of health professionals. A unique corpus such as this has great potential for researchers and practitioners as a means of studying highly sensitive concerns from a generation who have often been reluctant to consult practitioners, peers and others for personal health advice and information face to face (Suzuki and Calzo, 2004). The corpus approach to health communication affords an effective means of identifying the 'incremental effect' (Baker, 2006, p. 13) of patterns across large quantities of text, allowing the researcher and the language learner to discover linguistic routines which are liable to remain submerged in extensive data sets. The material in corpora such as this might well yield important and unexpected opportunities for advancing healthcare communication, both for second language learners of English in healthcare work, where a data-driven approach is gaining momentum, and in terms of a wider applicability in health communication learning as a whole.

Rietveld et al. (2004) note that the use of corpora has become common in language research over the last few decades. In many branches of linguistics, corpora provide core data for the development and testing of hypotheses. Equipped with such resources and with access to powerful software packages, the present-day researcher can explore the spoken word much more readily than in the early days of linguistics. Much of the classic work in language scholarship was performed without the benefit of the quantum leap in language awareness which corpus linguistics affords.

This example from a corpus linguistic study in healthcare is just one application of one kind of linguistic phenomenon in health. There are a great many more examples which we could have described. Fine-grained studies of interaction between practitioners and clients remain a popular topic, as do investigations of politeness phenomena, the language of medical records, the use of laughter and the role of interpreters. However, we felt it valuable to work through a single issue in some detail so the reader can see what may be yielded through the use of these techniques. As we have argued elsewhere (Brown et al., 2006; Crawford et al., 1998), the use of language is central to healthcare practice, and everything – from the whole life narrative to the minute details of conversational interaction – represents data from which a great deal can be gleaned for research and education.

Summary and Conclusions

We hope that in this chapter we have gone some way towards demonstrating the value of a narrative approach in healthcare. The narrative turn in health has been in full swing for three decades and there is now a great deal of material collected from a number of perspectives concerning a whole range of conditions. Some, such as cancer, have been studied extensively and others, such as healthcare-associated infections, have been subject to relatively little scrutiny. The focus of scholarship has shifted from the grand manifestos for the value of narrative medicine from Rita Charon or overall typologies of illness narrative from Arthur Frank to more detailed study of particular aspects of care and the patient journey. One of the lessons from literary study which has been widely applied in the healthcare field is that it is possible to detect regularly recurring patterns or forms in narrative, whether these be in terms of the beginning, middle and end stages, the moral lesson, such as the value of family life, or the resonance with earlier literary forms.

We have also examined how these narratives are not merely individual productions. They may well be co-constructed and co-produced. Study of the detail of clinical encounters shows how the interaction helps to produce narratives of a particular kind, jointly shaped by clinician and client. Moreover, narratives, causal scenarios, implicit working models and inferential structures enable people in family settings to collectively construct what may be troubling them and what might be the best course of action to take.

Linguistics has not hitherto been central to the medical humanities or the newer health humanities. However, we have tried to show, by way of our work on young people's problems written in to a health website, that it is possible to apply techniques from lexicography and second language learning such as corpus linguistics to elicit the patternings in larger data sets. This study also highlights that there is language to study in unexpected places which may provide insights into groups that have tended to be under-served by face to face healthcare.

Talking about one's health, or that of other people, is an enormously popular activity. However, it is important to be aware of what the narratives give us evidence of. They do not necessarily give us access directly to processes of sense-making, consciousness or mindedness on the part of the narrator. Neither do they provide direct knowledge of the social context in which the story took place. Despite their popularity we can make only quite modest claims about the evidence provided through narratives. However, their role in enriching the picture of health and illness, their potential to enhance understanding between practitioners and sufferers, their role in educating practitioners and their ability to build solidarity between sufferers themselves cannot be denied. The burgeoning field of narrative medicine within the health humanities is a testament to the desire to know something more than can be assessed simply through symptom checklists or investigation of the vital signs. The health humanities 'are not just a nice side dish of true medicine, but they are an indispensable part of patient oriented medicine' (Widder, 2004, p. 103).

5
Performing Arts and the Aesthetics of Health

The *performing arts* comprise an array of creative endeavours, in which artistic expression is conveyed through time, across a range of modalities and media, but which *directly involves the performer herself or himself*, within the artistic act, in some way (as opposed to creating an artefact, possibly to be subsequently shared, or displayed, with or without the artist physically present). Historically, the performing arts have played important social roles across human civilisations. They have served as a means of conveying beauty, perpetuating cultural myths and narratives, sanctioning moral values, containing and mastering psychological challenges within ritual spaces, provoking thought, and inspiring the imagination. While, in a popular sense, *performance* is typically understood as an act of a *performer* sharing artistic material with an *audience*, the constructs of 'performer' and 'audience' can actually be expanded to far broader domains of the overall human experience – most notably, to those domains encompassing the myriad dimensions of human health. This chapter will endeavour to explicate an understanding of the performing arts – specifically, the modalities of music, dance and drama – as *relational, aesthetic, temporal ways of being*, constituting practices of and pertaining to *health*.

Essential Attributes of the Performing Arts

As a foundation for understanding the performing arts as health practices, it is important to consider the essential attributes of the performing arts themselves – those features that qualify their fundamental nature, and what make them what they are, underlying their manifestations across a myriad of particular forms. For the purposes of framing the arguments presented here, three essential attributes of the performing arts are identified and summarised, consisting of their nature as *relational* (rooted in relationship), *aesthetic* (rooted in the qualitative integrity of experience and expression), and *temporal* (rooted in human time).

Performing Arts as Relational

Art, in any form, is a uniquely human phenomenon. As such, any essential attributes of the performing arts must be consistent with the essential attributes of being human. One of the most fundamental bases of humanity is *relationship*.

Ontologically, to be human means to be in relationship. On this point, Heidegger (1962) argues that existence is primarily a matter not of *what*, but of *who* beings (*Da-sein*) are, and that being means – without exception – *being-with* (*Mit-sein* or *Mit-da-sein*), or existence in relational (social) context. This fundamental, relational aspect of being human is *equiprimordial* to existence itself, and not bound to any particular conditions, including circumstantial aloneness, as Heidegger asserts:

> *Being-With* existentially determines Da-sein even when an other is not factically present and perceived.... This *Being-With* and the facticity of Being-With-One-Another are not based on the fact that several 'subjects' are physically there together. (p. 113)
>
> *Being-With* is an existential characteristic of Da-sein even when factically no Other is present-at-hand or perceived. Even Da-sein's Being-Alone is *Being-With* in the world. (pp. 156–157)

Nancy (2000) likewise asserts that being is always being-with, and that *I* always co-arises with *we*. Thus, existence is, essentially, co-existence. Buber (1971), in his treatise on the uniquely human, *I-Thou* encounter, submits that persons may regard one another on the level of person-ness, as mutual, biographical *subjects*, not merely as biological *objects* (the *I-It* encounter). Given the intrinsically relational nature of humanity on an existential level, encountering any individual person *as a person* (*who*), versus as a specimen the biological species called 'human' (*what*), means encountering humanity, collectively, on some level. Art, as a uniquely human phenomenon, is (like humanity) ontologically relational. The performing arts are, at their core, artistic *ways of being in relational context*. This relational context prevails, even in the circumstantial absence of an audience, such as when one encounters or performs music, dance or drama under private, solitary conditions. Thus, in a sense, insofar as the performing arts are situated in relational context, humanity is always the audience.

Moreover, just as being-in-relationship transcends the concreteness of physical body and observable behaviour, the relational nature of the performing arts transcends physical media and technical procedures. The performing arts, like persons, are located within the living contexts of shared, culturally situated, relational space and time. Thus, as ways of being-in-relationship, the performing arts cannot be reified or used as 'things', anymore than persons can be likewise objectified. By extension, like persons, the performing arts embody human *agency*, not subject to deterministic causality. It makes little or no sense to explain or predict the processes and impact of performing arts according to any generalisable, law-like, natural forces, independent of human values, meanings and identities. From a disciplinary perspective, therefore, the performing arts are generally better understood according to the tenets of the *humanities*, versus those of the *natural sciences*.

Performing Arts as Aesthetic

The performing arts, like any form of art, centrally concern the qualitative integrity of human experience and expression. Building upon the previous attribute, the performing arts may be understood as *relational, aesthetic, ways of being*.

Whether or not encountered as 'beautiful', the performing arts exist in relation to beauty-centred *values* such as creativity, imagination, playfulness, balance, coherence, meaningfulness, and so forth. Furthermore, there is no factually objective basis for appraising the artistic integrity of a given performed work, independent of human experience and expression, situated within socially negotiated, intersubjective contexts. Thus, a performed work is artistic to the extent that it is encountered and expressed as such and, like its relational dimensions, its aesthetic dimensions are best apprehended via the constructivist tenets of the humanities (versus natural science).

Evidence, in the form of prehistoric, archaeological artefacts and drawings, suggests that the aesthetic component of the performing arts has played a key role in human development, from the primordial dawn of human civilisation. Dissanayake (1992), citing such evidence as part of her thesis on *Homo Aestheticus*, asserts that the aesthetic dimension is inextricably a part of being human, and that it has always been central in the survival and continuity of the human species. Dissanayake (2009) further cites the *proto-aesthetic* dispositions of infants, who inter-respond with parents in artistically expressive ways, as acquiring developmental communicativeness. On a sociocultural level, DeNora (2007) contends that the performing arts (in this case, specifically with respect to the modality of music) are human acts of everyday, relational (or social) context, serving as *affordances* (opportunities) of human *resources* and social *capital* (in a sense different from reified objects of currency) which may be *appropriated* (in a sense different from manipulation and/or possession) by those who need it, all as part of the well-being of communities and cultures. Thus, they play a key role not only in human development, but also in human civilisation.

As is the case for persons, any given part of a performed artwork is only meaningful with respect to the whole (whether potential or actual) transcending the sum of its component parts, in relational context. What is a human hand, for example, independent of the life-world of the person who *performs* human acts with it? Likewise, what is an isolated note of music, an isolated gesture in a dance, or one isolated moment of a dramatic act, independent of how it inter-relates (or may inter-relate) to other elements, in its human context? Aesthetic experience, therefore, cannot be dissected in a reductionist manner. Moreover, while neuroanatomical correlates of aesthetic experience may be a phenomenon of interest to some, a person's entire history and life-world informs the nature of any given aesthetic encounter. Thus, any neuroanatomical correlates to the aesthetic dimensions of the performing arts are idiosyncratic to individual identities (another indication that the disciplinary 'home' of the performing arts is the humanities).

Performing Arts as Temporal

Performance is an act that unfolds in *time*; thus, all of the performing arts are *aesthetic acts that unfold in time*. Building upon the two previous attributes, the performing arts may be understood as *relational, aesthetic, temporal ways of being*.

The performing arts are not restricted to concrete, material time, unfolding in the sense of *chronos*, or the objective passing of 'clock' time, proceeding independently in its own right, as an absolute reference point for events. Rather, it unfolds more in the sense of *kairos*, or the inter-subjective passing of phenomenological, human time, consisting of meaningful events, proceeding in relational context, situated within the relativity of culture and history. According to Smith (1969), *chronos* is quantitative time, whereas *kairos* is qualitative time. In a sense, *chronos* is the 'what' of time, pertinent to the natural sciences, whereas *kairos* is the 'who' of time, pertinent to the humanities, and through which the performing arts unfold, relationally and aesthetically.

Time in the performing arts manifests as the pace in which meaningful events pass, within the work. This pace may be indicated in various ways. Music, for example, employs qualitative tempo markings (adagio, andante, allegro, etc.), aesthetic organisation of the pulse into meters and measures, aesthetic 'time-play' (e.g. rubato and fermata), and identification of temporal 'units' of musical meaning, such as phrases. These indicators are not meaningful on their own, but by virtue of their relationship to some greater, contextualised, aesthetic-temporal whole. The whole temporal form 'lives' though time, *teleologically*, perpetually incorporating both *where it has been*, and *where it is (or may be) going*, into any given present moment of the performance. The performing arts are not merely strings of disembodied, de-contextualised moments of stimuli. Chronologic time may be meaningful in the performing arts, but only to the extent that they play an artistic role as part of a larger structure unfolding in kairologic time (for example, when precise, mathematic quanta are employed in music, dance or drama as a very deliberate, *artistic* dimension of the work). However, it holds no intrinsic relevance in the performing arts, any more than does the measured volume of paint used on a canvas, or the number of words on a page of poetry.

Understanding Health Practices as Relational, Aesthetic and Temporal

The argument that the performing arts (as understood according to the above) constitute health practices rests upon the sub-argument that health practices can be understood as *ways of being-in-relationship, aesthetically, in time*.

The term *health* (Online Etymology Dictionary, n.d.) derives from *hāl* (Old English) and *kailo* (Proto-Indo-European) meaning 'whole'. Returning to these roots of the term, the construct of health as wholeness does not necessarily connote the idea of a singular, normative model of wellness, in which health is understood as proximity to a statistical norm, based upon biophysiological and behavioural indicators, independent of the relativity of individual contexts. Rather, health – as it pertains specifically to humanity – inextricably includes those attributes that are humanly relevant. It is a contextually relative, socially negotiated, lifelong, evolving phenomenon concerning actualisation of potentials at any given point during the course of one's life. Consistent with this distinction is Antonovsky's (1979, 1987) model of health that distinguishes (respectively) *pathogenesis* from *salutogenesis*.

Health, from a human perspective, therefore, can be understood as a way of being that is, like the performing arts, *relational, aesthetic* and *temporal*. It is relational, as it unfolds in social context; it is aesthetic, as the meaning of what 'counts' as being well is a matter of qualitative, inter-subjective negotiation; and it is temporal, in that health is a dynamic (not static) condition, unfolding over time, as does life, in humanly-relevant *kairos* (versus *chronos*). As beings who exist in relationship, persons are healthy to the extent that they are *relationally* well, or whole. That is, to the extent that their relational, situated identity and personal context provides them with opportunities to actualise their ever-shifting human potentials, and to the extent that they indeed act upon those opportunities that, in part, may give rise to new, greater ways of being-in-relationship. Human well-being is relevant to the extent that it concerns the qualitative integrity, or the *aesthetics*, of existence. The term 'wholeness', closely related to 'health', indicates not only that one possesses enough of one's own parts, but that there is meaningful coherence and beauty-centredness within one's being, *beyond* any particular parts, *in light of* present components and *in spite of* absent components. Moreover, the temporality of health (or *health-time*) can only be understood in terms of identity, and what health means within the biographical context of a person's lived experience, as it unfolds in time.

This idea of health paralleling the performing arts aligns well with Antonovsky's (1987) construct *sense of coherence*, or the sense of wholeness of one's self that affords one the capacity to manage the challenges of life and world. This idea also aligns well with the work of DeNora (2007), who asserts that health is something *performed* in situated, social context, including negotiation of values and among all of the life-worlds of the stakeholders. For DeNora, health comprises *performance* that someone *does* (i.e. via agency) as a relational being, as opposed to something done *to* or *for* someone as object. Health, like the performing arts, is understood as the work of appropriating the numerous affordances for health – affordances that, like any form of social capital, may or may not be distributed in socially egalitarian ways. Thus, for DeNora, health practices, as inherently sociocultural phenomena, are inherently political.

There is a relational-aesthetic-temporal dimension to every domain of human health and functioning, whether it concerns moving, thinking, communicating, feeling, or anything else. Each is humanly relevant only to the extent that it is, on some level, relational, aesthetic and temporal in nature. Figure 5.1 illustrates this dimension of health, across several basic domains of health (as examples).

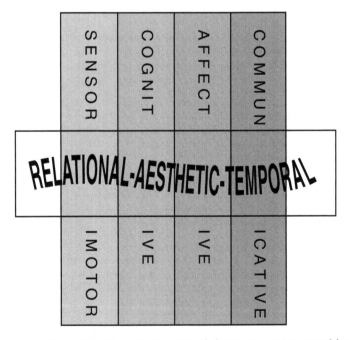

Figure 5.1 The relational-aesthetic-temporal dimension across several basic domains of health

Given an understanding of both health and the performing arts as relational-aesthetic-temporal phenomena, whenever and wherever the performing arts pertain to the matter of human well-being and wholeness, they may be understood as relational-aesthetic-temporal *health practices*. These practices serve a number of distinct purposes, three of which will be highlighted here: health *promotion*, health *communication* (including expression, education and discourse), and health *inquiry*. The performing arts for health *promotion* comprise practices of working together with others, for the purposes of helping to improve, maintain or restore health (this category of practice encompasses the *clinical* arts health disciplines, such as music, dance-movement, and drama therapies, but also includes practices that occur on the level of whole communities that may not typically be viewed as 'clinical' in any conventional sense). The performing arts for health *communication* encompasses the more specific practices of *expression*, or conveying (privately or publicly) experiences of health issues, healthcare, life surrounding health issues, etc., *education*, or conveying knowledge, skills and abilities pertinent to understanding health, and *discourse* or conversing about and/or formulating critique for social justice and pro-equality action pertaining to health issues. The performing arts for health *inquiry* encompass the practice of art-based research (Hervey, 2000; McNiff, 1998, 2008) concerning health. An elaboration upon the performing arts, understood as health practices, will be given in the section that follows, specifically in terms of three different performing arts modalities: music, dance and drama.

The Performing Arts as Health Practices: Three Different Modalities

Each modality of the performing arts constitutes a distinct mode of relational-aesthetic-temporal being. As such, each encompasses a distinct set of health practices. Here, the defining, essential characteristics of the modalities music, dance and drama will be identified, followed by examples of how each manifests as the practices of health promotion, health communication, and health inquiry.

Music

Music, at its essential core, consists of a way of being, relationally, aesthetically and temporally, in the most general sense. Therefore, music represents the 'root' performing arts modality, underpinning all of the others. Figure 5.2 shows a concentric circle diagram, illustrating the essence of music as relational, aesthetic, temporal being, comprising the 'root' essence of the performing arts.

There is archaeological evidence to suggest that music has been a part of human culture for over 30,000 years (Conard et al., 2009), and that it has been intimately tied to human health from prehistorical expressions of shamanism (Harvey and Wallis, 2007). Accordingly, Zuckerkandl (1956) developed the concept of *homo musicus*, which asserts that music is a property of humankind, inherent in *all* persons. Theory and research on phenomena such as *proto-musicality* (Dissanayake, 2001) and *communicative musicality* (Malloch and Trevarthan, 2010) demonstrate how the human capacities for affect, thought and language develop through everyday, pre-linguistic, musical exchanges of sound and feeling between infant and parent. Pertinent to health, this human primacy of music allows one to

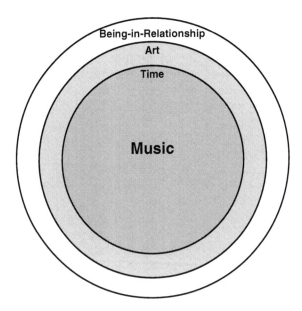

Figure 5.2 The essence of music as relational, aesthetic, temporal being – the 'root' essence of the performing arts

'hear' one's own potential for *becoming*, via the experience in music. Along these lines, Robbins (2005) has written:

> There is a lived and living affinity between what we call the 'laws of music' – in all their cultural diversity – and the totality of our spiritual, emotional, mental, and physical evolving. In this sense music as a conveyor of meaning in time might be said to mediate the historic, emergent dynamics of our past and continuing evolution. In some as yet indefinable way, the elements and expressive life of music speak of how we have come to be what and how we are. (p. 203)

Music is a culturally situated phenomenon that, in spite of certain common, shared attributes, is not so much one phenomenon, but many phenomena. What 'counts' as music varies from context to context; hence, the frequent use of the plural term 'musics'. Moreover, because music, as a temporal phenomenon (Pogoriloffsky, 2011), unfolds as participatory action-in-time, it has been conceptualised in verb form, as *musicing* (Elliott, 1995) or *musicking* (Small, 1998), both denoting music as a contextualised action (hereafter, the term will be spelled with the 'k'). These perspectives support the notion of music as an expression of human agency, and as a phenomenon located in social context and in humanity.

The concept of *play* is central in music, in both senses of the term: One may *play*, and *play in*, music. Music also involves *interplay*, or the relational component of music (between music, musicians, listeners, etc.). In play, there is freedom to express, while negotiating the boundaries of material, procedural and thematic 'givens'. Play is not merely casual, light-hearted fun (although such qualities may, at times, be present) – it is an organic, evolving process of relating and discovering, in which elements are encountered, engaged, synthesised and performed, in authentically meaningful ways. Play is driven by a person's agency and will, and often follows a somewhat meandering, nonlinear path, yet the results are of great human health relevance, beyond that which could ever be achieved through a rationalised, regimented experience. As Abrams (2010) contends:

> In the simple act of expanding one's capacities for musical experience and play in particular ways, beyond one's previous limits to

these capacities, one has shifted something fundamental about one's being, relevant to numerous other domains of health... Yet, at the same time, there is something in music that transcends those other domains. Just as any health domain cannot ultimately be reduced completely to any of the others, music as a health domain holds its own intrinsic legitimacy and meaningfulness *as health*, independently of what it signifies with respect to other domains. (online source)

Thus, the capacity for play is largely what characterises the relational, aesthetic, temporal dimension of health present in every domain of human health.

Music is typically understood as a performing art expressed through the physical medium of sound. While music may be expressed *through* or as *sound*, sound is not among the essential attributes of music itself. Just as no art form is bound to any concrete, physical medium, neither is music bound to sound (Abrams, 2011, 2012, 2013). Figure 5.3 shows the diagram with a partially overlapping circle representing sound, demonstrating how sound, while potentially present, is neither necessary nor sufficient in defining the core essence of music. From this perspective, musical sounds are not ultimately *about* the sounds themselves, but about ways of being. Zuckerkandl (1956) has written about how music cannot be found in sonic tones themselves, but rather in the aesthetic *to which they refer*, by virtue of their structural juxtaposition and sequencing. Moreover, it is notable that *soundless* components of music, such as rests or extended silences, can only signify anything musical by virtue of their juxtaposition within some larger, artistic context. The medieval philosopher Boethius (1989) made a related point long ago, distinguishing the construct *Musica Instrumentalis*, or the expression of music in sound, from *Musica Humana*, or the music of human existence itself. Importantly, *Musica Humana*, the fundamental basis for the more concrete *Musica Instrumentalis*, embodies the qualitative integrity of human being that may be understood as a particular dimension of *health* – specifically, the depth, coherence, meaningfulness and beauty expressed in aesthetically integrated movement, speech, thought, feeling, communication, and so forth – embodied in and manifesting across all domains of human health (Abrams, 2010, 2011, 2012). Given that music is not, itself, restricted to physical sound, persons who are unable to hear, who are averse to certain sounds (e.g. hyperacusis), or who are unable to process musical sound in conventional ways (e.g. amusia), are still equipped to apprehend and engage in music (Abrams, 2011).

Music as Health Promotion

Music as *health promotion* consists of practices with the general purpose of improving, maintaining or restoring human wholeness and well-being, in some capacity. These practices differ across characteristics such as their goals, applications (i.e. everyday, professional/clinical, self-help, etc.), ways of understanding music, ways of understanding persons, ideas about health, and so forth.

Stige (2002) provides a notion of one form of music as health promotion, *health musicking*, that combines the ideas of DeNora's (2007) health as situated performance and Small's (1998) music as contextualised action, into the assessment and application of health affordances of musical arenas, agendas, agents, activities and artefacts. Health musicking includes any practice where people use

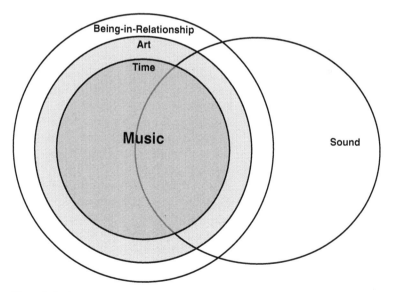

Figure 5.3 Sound, while potentially present, is neither necessary nor sufficient in defining the core essence of music

music experiences to create meaning and coherence in states and times of adversity (Bonde, 2011), and can include activity that occurs both within and beyond the therapy room (Stige, 2002). An example of music as health promotion – in this case, of *health musicking* – is described by Clift and Hancox (2010), pertaining to their work on the inherent health-promoting benefits of singing together in a community choir (addressing physiological, cognitive/educational, emotional and social domains). Stige writes about another form of music as health promotion, *music therapy*, as one, specific form of health musicking. He defines it as 'situated health musicking in a planned process of collaboration between client and therapist' (Stige, 2002, p. 200). Proctor (2004) offers an account of *community music therapy* as therapeutic redistribution of music capital (in the sense of empowering affordances and appropriations) for mental health.

Music as Health Communication

Music, as a relational phenomenon, embodies numerous communicative capacities. As already described here, *communicative musicality* (Malloch and Trevarthan, 2010) is one of the most primal forms of human interaction. Across the lifespan, and across society, music can express, educate about, and generate discourse about health in numerous ways. As expression, it can convey the experience of struggles with health issues, such as that of women and eating disorders featured in the song *Fatso*, as performed by The Story (Brooke and Kimball, 1993), or the experience of addiction featured in the song *Chet Baker's Unsung Swan Song*, as performed by David Wilcox (1994). As education, it can convey health-based information, such as songs composed and performed in the context of a health education programme in Uganda, designed to engender knowledge about teen pregnancy, HIV, and other sexually transmitted infections (Alford et al., 2005). As discourse, it can engage conversation and critique about the societal forces that perpetuate child abuse conveyed in *Luka*, as performed by Suzanne Vega (1987), or rape culture depicted in the song *Me and a Gun*, as performed by Tori Amos (1991).

Music as Health Inquiry

Music as health inquiry means one particular modality through which *art-based research* may be practised. Art-based research is, essentially, an artistic way of exploring and coming to know (in an epistemological sense) a given phenomenon of interest. As McNiff (2008) frames it:

> Art-based research can be defined as the systematic use of the artistic process, the actual making of artistic expressions in all of the different forms of the arts, as a primary way of understanding and examining experience by both researchers and the people that they involve in their studies. (p. 29)

On the topic of health, art-based research using music has been employed to explore and understand phenomena such as trauma and addiction (Austin, 2004).

Dance

Dance, at its essential core, consists of a way of being, relationally, aesthetically and temporally, like music; however, dance occurs specifically in *corporal* (body) *space*. Corporal space is not merely the concreteness of a biological space. It is the space of physical self as situated in the context of individual and collective human identity. In other words, beyond the *what* of some physiological organism, it is the *who* of *someone's* body. It is in this *situatedness* of body – this corporal *way of being* – where the corporal dimension of dance is located; thus, like any art, dance is not bound to material media. Like *Musica Humana*, this principle can be conceptualised as *Chorea Humana*. Therefore, the component of corporal space relevant to dance as a performing arts modality is that which intersects the relational, the aesthetic and the temporal realms, and it is this very intersection that differentiates dance from the more general essence of music. Figure 5.4 shows a concentric circle diagram defining the essence of dance as a relational, aesthetic, temporal, corporal way of being.

As is the case with music, dance long pre-dates recorded history and, since its inception, has been an important part of ceremony, sacrament, rites of passage, celebration, and, pertinent to health, shamanic healing ritual (Kassing, 2007). Dance ranges from functional movement (e.g. folk dance), to athletic movement (e.g. gymnastics, ice skating, etc.), to formal art dance (e.g. ballet). Particular definitions and boundaries around what 'counts' as dance vary according to a given culture's particular set of aesthetic and moral sensibilities.

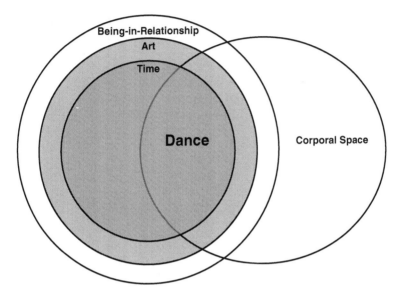

Figure 5.4   The essence of dance as a relational, aesthetic, temporal, corporal way of being

Like music, the *play* dimension of dance is central. Within the 'givens' of a choreographed dance, there remains room for play and interplay among the various elements of the choreography. Dance occupies a significant role in everyday life as well – for example, in social metaphors such as 'dance' in the sense of interpersonal negotiation and reciprocity, 'dancing around an issue' as social evasion, feeling 'moved' as emotional impact, or feeling 'in step' or 'out of step' in the sense of social harmony or disharmony (respectively). Pertinent to health, dance can embody capacities of personal presence, motor skill, gestural communicativeness, negotiation of relative physical power and strength, etc.

Dance as Health Promotion

Dance as *health promotion* consists of practices with the general purpose of improving, maintaining or restoring human wholeness and well-being, in some capacity. Like music, these practices differ across characteristics such as their goals, applications, and ways of regarding dance, persons and health. Examples include a dance and movement programme to improve quality of life for breast cancer survivors (Sandel et al., 2005) and a dance/movement therapy programme to address the special needs of young children with specific disorders (e.g. autism spectrum, attachment, etc.) (Tortora, 2009).

Dance as Health Communication

Dance, like music, is highly communicative. It is human thought and feeling expressed in the form of structured, aesthetic movement comprising a system of communicative rules, applicable to a variety of social situations (Hanna, 1987), and can express, educate about, and generate discourse about health, in a number of ways. As expression, it can publicly convey the experience of life-threatening illness, as was accomplished in a series of performances about cancer by the OnStage Dance Company (2012). Also concerning cancer, dance, as education, can raise consciousness about the illness. This was largely the intention of Texas-based choreographer and dancer Sharon Marroquín (diagnosed with breast cancer in 2010), in her work, 'The materiality of impermanence' (2012). As discourse, it can challenge public assumptions about mental illness, as California-based choreographer Hazel Clark (2013) accomplished via her piece, 'A question that sometimes drives me hazy: Am I, or are the others crazy?' The performance included a guest speaker from the National Alliance for Mental Illness.

Dance as Health Inquiry

Dance, like music, can serve as an artistic way of knowing in the process and outcomes of health-based research inquiry. For example, Boydell (2011) conducted art-based qualitative health research in which care during first episode psychosis was explored via music, allowing the research team to address the visceral, emotional and visual aspects of the research, not otherwise available in more conventional research. As another example, Rutledge (2004) utilised creative dance experiences in the process of inquiring into the phenomenon of *surrender*, through which the project participants explored and negotiated ideas about the subject matter. The research process drew from interpretive phenomenological and art-based methodologies, and findings carried implications for better understanding human personal development.

Drama

Drama, at its essential core, consists of a way of being, relationally, aesthetically and temporally, like music; however, drama occurs specifically in *narrative* (i.e. *stories*, whether based upon fictional or nonfictional constructions). Stories are inherently human, as narrative is a central way in which human beings understand their lives, both as individual persons, and as collective peoples (co-constructed within communities and/or cultures). Narrative is, therefore, always a way of being-in-relationship, and is always (in some way) socially situated. However, it is not always an art form, as it often serves a purely functional, non-aesthetic role. Moreover, it is not always a temporal form, as there are ways in which narrative can be embodied in static space, such as in paintings, sculptures or tableaus (the lattermost representing, in a sense, a *dance-like* phenomenon, existing outside of time). Therefore, the component of narrative relevant to drama as a performing arts modality is that which intersects both the aesthetic and the temporal realms, and it is this very intersection that differentiates drama from the more general essence of music. Figure 5.5

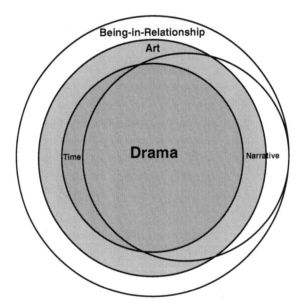

Figure 5.5   The essence of drama as a relational, aesthetic, temporal, narrative way of being

shows a concentric circle diagram defining the essence of drama as a relational, aesthetic, temporal, narrative way of being. It is worthy of note that, according to this model, whenever music or dance involve narrative components, they are actually forms of drama, whether or not popularly characterised as such.

Drama is typically understood as a form expressed through corporal (body) space on the stage, and through the physical medium of sound – most often, verbal monologue and dialogue, but also musical sound, as in the cases of opera and musical theatre, wherein music plays an integral role in conveying and accompanying dramatic texts, or Japanese *Noh*, wherein musical sound accompaniment underscores text and/or action. However, there are cases of *spaceless* drama, such as that conveyed via sound alone (e.g. radio drama), and *soundless* drama, such as pantomime, or otherwise lengthy periods of silent, textless narrative. Thus, drama may be expressed *through* stage and/or sound, yet drama is not bound to either concrete, physical medium, as an essential, defining element. Like *Musica Humana* and *Chorea Humana*, this principle can be conceptualised as *Drama Humana*. Figure 5.6 shows the diagram with partially overlapping circles representing corporal space and sound, demonstrating how both, while potentially present, are neither necessary nor sufficient in defining the core essence of drama.

As is the case with both music and dance, drama likely has roots in prehistoric society. Its primary history, however, is associated with the Classical period. The term 'drama' derives from the Ancient Greek verb 'to act', and was traditionally structured according to collaborative modes of production (i.e. involving more than one person), as well as collective forms of reception (i.e. an audience) (Pfister, 1977). The two masks associated with drama – symbols of the Ancient Greek muses *Thalia* and *Melpomene* – represent a distinction between the two traditional, primary theatrical genres of comedy and tragedy, respectively. Although drama may be based upon a text, it is not primarily about the verbal content of the words; rather, it is about the underlying action, or the dramatic *ways of being*. Fergusson (1968), in support of this principle, writes:

> A drama, as distinguished from a lyric, is not primarily a composition in the verbal medium; the words result, as one might put it, from the underlying structure of incident and character. As Aristotle remarks, 'the poet, or "maker" should be the maker of

plots rather than of verses; since he is a poet because he imitates, and what he imitates are actions'. (Idea #8)

Like both music and dance, there is a 'play' dimension in drama, as implied by the manner in which the term *play* denotes a dramatic work.

Pertinent to health, a number of scholars have conceptualised health in *dramaturgical* terms, as health performance in social

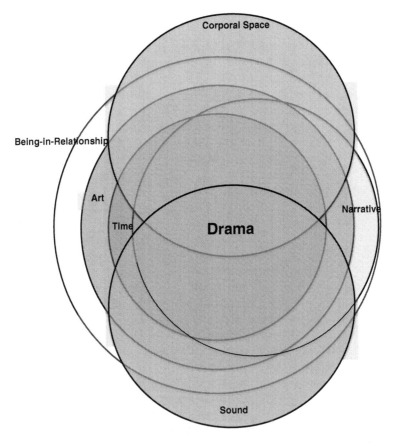

Figure 5.6 Corporal space and sound, while potentially present, are neither necessary nor sufficient in defining the core essence of drama

context (e.g. Aldridge, 1996, 2004; DeNora, 2000, 2007; Ruud, 1998; Stige, 2012). As a manifestation of this principle, everyday human discourse is replete with social metaphors tied to drama, and which are relevant to health and well-being. The term 'drama' itself can refer to the inflation of a given situation's significance, or behaviour that communicates inflated self-significance and disproportionate needs driven by narcissism or insecurity. 'Theatrics', for example, can signify a form of passive-aggressive attention-seeking behaviour. 'Drama queen' is used in a related way, with the added connotation of derogatory, feminine stereotypy. 'Acting' can signify either the dynamic exercise of everyday, human agency, or can invoke a judgemental reference to the fictional component of drama in appraising another's authenticity (i.e. it is 'all just an act'). 'Acting out' signifies the externalisation of internal, emotional conflict, often in socially inappropriate ways. 'Stage' can refer, as a verb, to planning, organising and carrying out an act for public effect, often for the benefit of a particular group of stakeholders (i.e. 'staging a protest'). It can also refer to a phase of a process, including human development. Shakespeare makes a dual reference to this term as both place (dramatic venue) and time (human lifespan) in the monologue from *As You Like It*, beginning with the famous line, 'All the world's a stage'.

Drama as Health Promotion

Drama as *health promotion* consists of practices with the general purpose of improving, maintaining or restoring human wholeness and well-being, in some capacity. Like both music and dance, these practices differ across characteristics such as their goals, applications, and ways of regarding drama, persons and health. Drama therapy, for example, helps people with emotional and disability-related needs via dramatic processes including role-play, enaction (scripted or improvisational), puppets, masks, storytelling, rituals, games, and so forth (Langley, 2006). An example is the application of dramatherapy in the neuro-trauma recovery room (McKenna and Haste, 1999).

Drama as Health Communication

Drama, like both music and dance, is centrally about communication, and conveys human stories in a myriad of forms. Thus, it too can express, educate about, and generate discourse about health, in a number of ways. As expression, it can convey the struggles among intellect, emotions and relationships while dying from terminal forms of illness, such as is conveyed in the play *Wit* (Edson, 1995). As education, a programme such as is described in the *Life Drama Project* (Baldwin, 2010), based in Papua New Guinea, applied theatre processes can incorporate cultural performativity, creativity and aesthetics in order to achieve the educational goal of helping the public understand the emotionally contradictory messages surrounding the prevalence and prevention of diseases such as HIV. As discourse, it can address the controversial topic of agency, autonomy and relationships in major healthcare decision-making, such as is illustrated in the plays *Whose Life Is It Anyway?* (Clark, 1972), in which a paralysed sculptor engages with others concerning his individual right to euthanasia, and *Mercy Killers* (Milligan, 2012), in which a man strives to care for and protect his critically ill wife, while struggling to navigate the dysfunction of the US healthcare system.

Drama as Health Inquiry

Drama, like both music and dance, can serve as an artistic way of knowing in the process and outcomes of health-based research inquiry. For example, Rossiter et al. (2008) utilised theatre as a tool for analysis and knowledge transfer, data transformation, and presentation of findings in health research. Specifically, they utilised ethnodrama, in which interview transcripts, field notes from participant observation, journals, documents and statistics are incorporated into a dramatic play script, and subsequently staged as a live, public theatre performance (Given, 2008). As another example, Mienczakowski (1999), drawing upon the work of his research team (Rolfe et al., 1995), created a play embodying struggles of persons with schizophrenia, as well as a play based upon the experiences of alcoholics who have undergone detoxification within an institution. Both were utilised in order to illuminate the nature of the subject matters, and both were performed by student actors and student nurses, for audiences consisting of research informants, students and healthcare professionals.

Summary and Conclusions

The prevailing healthcare culture and climate is generally oriented around a *monological* (versus *dialogical*) world-view based upon

principles of positivism and natural science. As such, it does not typically consider situated realities and negotiated meanings, and rarely
acknowledges the human primacy of *being-in-relationship*. Health is
generally understood as a physiological or behavioural fact, independent of the multidimensionality and relativity of social context.
And, when context *is* considered, it is typically regarded as a set of
variables, and still part of the same, technical chain of causality. To
a large extent, the behavioural and social sciences operate within a
natural science orientation, wherein the performing arts are considered valuable to the extent that they, as technical procedures, demonstrate a measurable, statistically predictable impact upon health.
Questions such as 'How well does "it" work?' and 'How well does "all
of this" work together?' prevail. By contrast, questions from a health
humanities framework, such as 'How well do "I" work?' (concerning
human locus of agency) or 'How well do "we" all work, together?'
(concerning the collective agency of a community or culture) are
usually not regarded as particularly relevant.

From a pragmatic standpoint, then, how is one to demonstrate
the value of a humanities-based understanding of the performing
arts, and the role it can play as part of health-centred endeavours?
It would be disingenuous for health-based performing artists with a
health humanities orientation to assimilate, thereby relinquishing
the unique contribution the health humanities perspective on the
performing arts can offer. Likewise, it would be self-defeating for
health-based performing artists to isolate, thereby remaining in a
marginalised position relative to the resources they need in order to
advance and succeed.

Perhaps it would be helpful to adopt multiple perspectives, each
representing part of a larger, inclusive, integral framework. The field
of music therapy, for example, has recognised a number of distinct
ways of understanding evidence based practice, and how each plays
a unique role within the larger scope of the field (Abrams, 2010).
While science contributes ways of knowing as technical causality and
prediction, the humanities can contribute ways of knowing as contexts, dialogue, and negotiated meanings. While the value of the former is typically considered a given, it is incumbent upon the latter to
demonstrate the mutuality of this relationship, and that the humanities perspective can contribute a vital framework that can better
serve all stakeholders by addressing the contexts *in which health is*

performed, therefore engendering an environment facilitating even *better scientific practices*. As a part of this mutuality and integral thinking, quality advocacy, education and diplomacy are necessary, and it is important to promote a characterisation of the performing arts as something beyond an entertainment commodity, and a characterisation of the health humanities as a paradigm home for real practices – not merely as an elite, intellectual, academic exercise.

From an economic standpoint, in a system that tends to assign value according to deterministic outcomes, via dose–response models and statistical, actuary computation (supportable by evidence generated by such procedures as the randomised controlled trial), an understanding of health practices that locate outcomes with the agency of persons and their performance of art may understandably represent a 'hard sell'. The prospect of monetising and allocating resources to the establishment of opportunity (versus assurance of controlled outcome), that may or may not be utilised by a given health service user, may be cause for hesitation. It is imperative to demonstrate the inherent and irreplaceable value in allocating resources to empowering service users and other stakeholders in the healthcare community with their own responsibility for utilising the opportunities established via the performing arts, in their various forms and for their various purposes.

Finally, from a socio-political standpoint, elevating an understanding of both the performing arts and health to *ways of being* establishes them as human resources and affordances to be appropriated in the interest of improving the human condition, in large part via addressing matters of equality and social justice surrounding health practices. This understanding can normalise the practice of aestheticising not only space (physical surroundings), but time (relational, human, *kairos*) in health-centred endeavours, thus better distributing aesthetic capital in the lives of all stakeholders, in mutually beneficial ways. This shift in understanding can help raise public awareness about the struggles and triumphs of those involved in health-centred work in ways that, unlike verbal discourse alone, can preserve the true morphicity (lived sense, contour, etc.) of these experiences. In addition, it can help unite the disciplines of arts and health which, when working in synergy, can enrich one another for the benefit of individuals, communities and society.

Whether pragmatic, economic or socio-political, the challenges of understanding the performing arts as health practices (from a health humanities perspective) must be accompanied by pertinent ethical considerations. What, for example, are the risk-to-benefit ratios when engaging individuals and communities via performing arts for the purposes of health promotion, health communication, and health inquiry? For example, in certain forms of health inquiry, is it possible that participants 'performing' health issues may experience certain forms of re-traumatisation or re-symptomisation? (Boydell et al., 2012). Fortunately, ethics itself is fundamentally a humanity and, thus, ethical thinking in implementing performing arts as health practices should come naturally, with relative ease, for the practitioners. Of course, a community of peers, through mutual contribution and negotiation, can only improve the ethical integrity of any projects promoting any thought and work in this area.

6
Visual Art and Transformation

There is growing evidence which supports the therapeutic utility of visual art. In this chapter visual art is referred to interchangeably as art or visual art. This includes work on neuroaesthetics, art as therapy, art as an educational tool, and art used to enhance clinical and public environments. These will be considered in turn with reference to three case studies which illustrate the wider utility of visual art in healthcare.

For most humans vision is their dominant sense, with 80 per cent of information about the world around us coming from visual stimuli and half of the brain cortex used for visual processing (Snowden et al., 2006). Early reports document the therapeutic benefits of art for example to facilitate communication and for 'spiritual regeneration' (Adamson, 1984; Carey, 2006). It is known that as early as the Upper Paleolithic through Mesolithic periods humans were engaged in producing cave paintings, beadwork and figurines. An abstract stone carving dating from 70,000 years ago found in South Africa suggests that art making was a part of human existence even earlier (BBC, 2002). There is a long tradition of art as foundational to culture and artistic practices tend to be ritualised, curated and held in high esteem, hence having potential therapeutic benefits individually and collectively.

The health-enhancing qualities of art derive from a number of sources. Colour, shape and form are known to impact on mood, reminiscence and attention, and galleries and museums are high status institutions, viewed as repositories of culture, history and invention. The creation of art involves a process which includes technique, intellect and engagement. The end product, or artwork, may take a number of different forms, for example painting, installation, sculpture, film or photograph. All these forms have in common an expression of the artist and, if curated and exhibited, the potential to alter physical environments and impact on an audience both cognitively and emotionally.

The aesthetic qualities of art have the ability to act upon mood and can enhance environments, having an immediate impact as well as a longer-term legacy. Art conveys therapeutic benefits for the maker and the viewer and art viewing can be experienced as a solitary pastime or communally through discussion and contemplation, thus giving it utility in a variety of formats.

Despite their potential health benefits the visual arts have historically been considered an elitist pastime (Efland, 1990) linked to Enlightenment principles of aesthetics which feature the educated and upper classes 'regarding' cultural objects in privileged and rarefied environments. Traditionally artistic and cultural artefacts have been reviewed, researched and curated by art historians and cultural theorists. This means that the potential therapeutic benefits of visual art have not been fully explored. More recently, however, interdisciplinary work has pointed to the evolutionary, social and community benefits of art – for example, art shared through participatory and socially engaged practice, also called community arts, as a means to connect individuals and alleviate social exclusion. The re-evaluation of artistic outputs by the untrained artist in the field of outsider art is another example of the area widening from a traditional art historical and cultural studies approach to one that encompasses health perspectives. This chapter assesses the contribution that visual arts are making to health and healthcare currently and addresses the role of this field within the health humanities in future.

Receptive Consumption: Viewing Art

The field of neuroaesthetics concerns the brain's response to art by examining the neural processes that occur when viewing and by exploring how art functions to evoke human responses (Zeki, 2011). Although beyond the remit of this chapter it should be noted that the field of neuroaesthetics is grounded in Eurocentric notions of aesthetics critiqued above, evolutionary psychology, and theories of emotion which neglect wider social and cultural practices (Brown and Dissanayake, 2009). Artwork has an affective response on the viewer via several routes; for example, the artist presents a narrative, or uses colour, form or line to arouse emotion. Viewers display a preference for elements such as symmetry which are thought to have an evolutionary basis as human beings who are symmetrical are perceived as healthy and therefore reproductively optimal. Diffuse, conceptual or abstract art may evoke a sense of fear which is related to uncertainty and disorientation, harking back to basic survival instincts. Individuals typically display a preference for artwork that is both complex and technically proficient. Artwork like this can have a powerful impact, by inducing an array of emotions or meta-emotions (Noy and Noy-Sharav, 2013).

Artists often focus on the 'essence' of something familiar and then extend or amplify it, thus causing arousal in the viewer – for example, Picasso's Cubist depictions of the female form. This creates a 'peak shift' which means that the brain is stimulated when it sees something recognisable which is then exaggerated to become like a caricature (Ramachandran and Hirstein, 1999). The pleasure derived from art viewing may be seen as a 'self-actualising' experience according to Maslow's hierarchy of needs (Maslow, 1954). In this hierarchy Maslow posits that all humans require their basic physiological and safety needs to be met, that is, food, shelter and warmth are required for survival. Once these basic needs are satisfied individuals can begin to reach 'higher' domains such as social relationships, self-esteem and education. Self-actualising experiences are those which relate to pleasure and realising one's potential, for example creative expression. Art is potentially therapeutic as it provides stimulation and pleasure at the point of creation, in its completion, and in the pleasure artistic outputs can bring to viewers.

Art as Communication

Visual art plays a strong role in communicating information. This may be figurative (literal) or in abstraction but whatever the style art is able to convey information that is complex, sensitive, distressing and emotive. Art uses a spatial matrix which enables numerous ideas to be expressed simultaneously, unlike the typically linear mode of verbal expression (Rubin, 2005). Dissanayake's writing on the biological and cultural aspects of art notes the relational aspects of art which helps to explain both the origins of art and its potency (2000). This acknowledges that art is part of our histories and is typically communicative and ceremonial. Take for example Goya's representations of the horrors of war, including violence, maiming and death, in his 19th-century series 'The Disasters of War', or Hogarth's 18th-century series 'The Rake's Progress' portraying a young man's descent into disrepute and madness. Both of these examples showcase the potential of art to depict complex issues simultaneously – in this case historical events and institutional practices, and aspects of the human condition such as depravity, degeneration, illness, death and dying. Visual art may also communicate the experience of illness – for example, the artist William Utermohlen's (1933–2007) documentation of dementia in a series of self-portraits after receiving the diagnosis of Alzheimer's disease. This series serves to illustrate a shift in his identity and his artistic style from figurative towards abstraction. As well as documenting his physical decline the series evokes a sense of confusion and alienation as his cognitive demise progresses, the work becoming more fractured and incoherent hence demonstrating the function of the spatial matrix. One may argue that looking at these images provides a more powerful rendering of the condition of dementia than a verbal description alone. This is especially the case with mental illness which cannot be easily 'seen'. In Utermohlen's case his communication is multi-faceted as he is both grappling with and documenting his condition as well as sharing the experience with others and raising awareness of dementia more widely.

Recently there has been development of art viewing programmes aiming to harness some of the benefits described above. Art viewing can be seen as analogous to a therapeutic encounter as it includes processes such as externalisation of problems, verbalising complex emotions, and an educational dimension (Roberts et al., 2011). An art viewing programme developed for people with dementia indicated that the activity stimulated mood, memory and cognition (Eekelaar et al., 2012) and another found that art viewing facilitated identity construction in older people (Newman et al., 2012). The variety of outcomes are indicative of the complexity of cognitive and interpersonal processes happening within the interventions. This is one difficulty in measuring the worth of such programmes and one which has challenged the published research to date.

Art as Therapy: Healing through Creativity

There is a long history of the use of artistic activity in healthcare. Art has been widely used as a pastime in clinical environments but developed more specific aims within fields such as mental health care. For example, it was used in asylums in the 19th century in an attempt to diagnose illness and patients were known to use the most crude materials available like toilet paper and matchsticks in their urge to produce artistic work. Creative activities such as basket weaving and carpentry were thought to be therapeutic for people who had experienced trauma, such as those returning from the Great War in the early 20th century (BBC, 2014). In 1946 Edward Adamson was appointed as an artist at the Netherne Psychiatric Hospital in Surrey, UK. There he established art workshops for patients and pioneered art as therapy. He is acknowledged as the forefather of art therapy and was an advocate for the utility of artistic expression in recovery from mental ill health. In his words artistic expression had 'the ability to heal' (Adamson, 1984, p. 8). The book *Healing Arts* (Hogan, 2001) charts the origins of art therapy and the connections between art from the asylum and wider artistic circles such as the Surrealists.

Artistic engagement is a powerful mode of expression in healthcare, especially where the artist may have problems in communication or where painful or complex experiences are narrated (Malchiodi, 2006). It is therefore often used as part of art therapy – for example, where individuals have experienced abuse or with those who may have difficulty communicating, such as children. Artistic expression can also reveal clues about an individual's mental state which provides important and relevant clinical information for health professionals (Demenaga and Jackson, 2010). Despite this the research evidence for such work lacks robustness. Standardised biomedical modes of measurement often fail to find any impact – for example, a randomised controlled trial comparing group art therapy with a control activity group and a group receiving usual care for individuals with a diagnosis of schizophrenia found no difference in outcomes in the three groups (Crawford et al., 2012).

Creative Practice: Making Art

Building upon the benefits of art viewing there is more recent interest in the potential of art making to convey health benefits. Research evidence suggests that making art improves attention, memory and communication (e.g. Camic et al., 2013; Reynolds, 2010). Those actively engaged in making art often refer to a 'flow' state, that is a condition of peak performance conducive to well-being. This involves the synergy of physical and psychological functioning, likened to a transcendent, ecstatic condition of effortless yet focused and optimal performance (Csikszentmihalyi, 1997). When art making is practised as a collective activity, social benefits such as decreasing isolation and building networks of support are reported (Camic et al., 2013). Participatory arts projects engaging marginalised or diverse groups of individuals may have wider aims such as building communities and social inclusion. In such activities the creation of artwork may be viewed as a by-product of wider social processes (Stickley and Duncan, 2010). Such projects foreground the collective experiences of participants as a form of individual and community action and it is notable that aesthetic outcomes may be a lesser priority than the experience shared by the group (Sánchez Camus, 2009).

Creative Dissemination

Recognising that works of visual art are typically celebrated as cultural artefacts suggests that work produced within art-making programmes can have utility beyond the therapeutic encounter. Art making can become a transformative and empowering process, as illustrated in Case Study 6.1. This is compatible with a social model of disability which focuses upon structural inequality rather than individual impairment. Without entering philosophical debates about the 'quality' of such outputs or their ethical status, such work can be exhibited publicity for appraisal, critique and possibly sale. For example, the outsider art field embraces work produced by artists who are largely untrained and therefore unconstrained by convention and who often have severe health challenges such as chronic mental health problems or learning difficulties. Interest in creative work by the untrained gained prominence with the artist Jean Dubuffet who first used the term Art Brut in 1945, referring to work that has a 'purity' in existing outside of or peripheral to the mainstream. In 1972 the art historian Roger Cardinal coined the term 'outsider art' for this type of work. Since then the outsider art field has grown and become so well established that there are numerous galleries across the world specialising in this type of work and commercial art fairs

Case Study 6.1   *Art as transformation*

Engagement with artistic practice can be transformative at an individual and societal level, as one study of people with mental health problems revealed (Visholm, 2010). Four individuals submitting work to an exhibition on mental health issues were interviewed in depth about their mental health, their creative practice and the impact it had on them. A phenomenological approach was taken to the analysis of textual interview data. The results identify the ability of art to communicate the personal and intimate in private spheres such as therapeutic encounters and also to transcend boundaries by publicly highlighting the power of artwork to heal personally and to act socially, culturally and in some cases politically in raising issues about mental health problems. Artwork was both consciously and unconsciously used to counteract stigma about mental illness and to create new identities for those who experienced disempowerment as a result of their ill health. As one participant 'Max' expressed:

Art offers a different sort of vocabulary, you can express things in art that you can't in words.

Another participant 'Sarah' describes the process involved in directly processing mental illness and moving towards self-realisation:

The first painting was about therapy for me and understanding the mess and trying to make sense of it, the second one was about understanding who I really am.

selling work by untrained creators, some of whom have achieved considerable success and recognition by art critics.

Art as Education: Interdisciplinary Excursions in Healthcare Teaching with Visual Art

As Freedman points out, inclusion of visual culture in curricula cultivates not only personal enrichment but also cultural identity and political ideology (Freedman, 2003). Alongside subjects including literature and philosophy, visual art has been utilised as part of the medical humanities which aims to inculcate physicians and medical students with holistic values, in particular foregrounding the perspective of the patient and nurturing the personal development of the physician. The medical humanities is an established field of endeavour in the US and the UK although disciplines outside medicine have had lesser focus, an issue being redressed through this volume and the activities of its authors.

It is recognised that interdisciplinary teaching can encourage healthcare students to adopt a holistic approach to patient care, one which foregrounds patient experience and encourages empathy. Interprofessional projects can lead to team building and an appreciation for different approaches and techniques, important skills for students who will work in multi-disciplinary teams post-qualification. Visual art can provide an alternative narrative, particularly where patients may find it difficult to communicate or where illnesses are hard to articulate. It is therefore an ideal modality to present emotional or complex information which may underpin individual experiences of illness and recovery. Viewing contemporary art is noted to improve observational skills in the training of medical students (Schaff et al., 2011) and a project using artists to teach alongside anatomists in the study of anatomy led to medical students developing an increased appreciation of the human form, for example noticing the differing hues of the skin (Tischler et al., 2011).

Artistic training has applicability beyond medicine as in both medical and nursing students it is noted to enhance empathy and observation, thus benefitting the development of clinical skills (Collett and McLachlan, 2005; Frei et al., 2010; Tischler et al., 2010). Visual arts approaches are aligned with patient-centredness, an approach which places patients at the heart of healthcare. Healthcare professionals practising in a patient-centred way encourage patients to be active and equal decision-makers in their care. It has also been suggested that such courses, as well as increasing students' level of artistic skill, can encourage them to embrace a broader world-view rather than being constrained by the scientific domain (Phillips, 2000). Beyond clinical practice such training benefits the individual by nurturing their own creativity and providing respite from stressful vocational practice (Tischler et al., 2011).

Aesthetic Environments: Art and Spaces

Visual art is perhaps unique amongst the humanities disciplines in its ability to transform environments using colour, pattern, texture and scale. It is recognised that environmental contexts are important in healthcare and can impact on mood and morale. A number of projects have utilised visual art to enhance clinical environments – for example 'Paintings in Hospitals', a charity which loans artworks to healthcare establishments (Paintings in Hospitals, 2014) – and patients in palliative care may be encouraged to bring objects such as pictures and quilts from home to 'soften' the clinical environment (Campbell, 2012). Staricoff (2004) reported that use of artwork in this way not only improved the environment but helped to reduce anxiety and depression, as well as the length of hospital stay, and boosted staff morale. Although this chapter does not focus on design of clinical environments, a case could be made for institutions such as hospitals being considered as 'cultural resources' (MacNaughton, 2007) as they can provide therapeutic spaces through inclusion of art and other creative practices and impact on populations with particular health challenges. These issues tend to take a back seat in a publicly funded healthcare system such as the National Health Service (NHS) where functionality, infection control and cost dominate the agenda. Yet if attractive design can be shown to be cost-effective – for example leading to shorter stays – then a case can be made for incorporating art in clinical environments. Research indicates that the aesthetic environment is important to patients in hospital, and a study of elderly people – who represent the largest group of the population using healthcare – suggested that receptive arts were more important when illness was acute, with participative activities of more interest in rehabilitative and recovery phases of illness (Moss and O'Neill, 2014).

Cultural Spaces as Healthcare Venues

Cultural institutions such as art galleries and museums are beginning to explore collaboration with healthcare researchers and organisations. Such institutions are often publicly or philanthropically funded and have a remit to engage with the general population and to serve the public good. This is achieved through education, learning or integrated programmes delivered alongside high quality art for consumption. Targeting multiple audiences has a democratising effect as it encourages non-traditional visitors into venues which are traditionally and currently the preserve of the middle and upper classes (Hanquinet, 2013). Galleries have therapeutic qualities which have not been fully exploited – for example, they are often quiet and contemplative. These may be utilised as 'non-clinical' environments which offer a contrast to healthcare venues as they are community based, accessible and non-stigmatising. Facilitating access to these venues can enhance social and cultural capital in marginalised groups (Goulding, 2013). Use of galleries and museums in this way creates alternative spaces for the public to use both to manage health issues and to enhance well-being. Beyond galleries non-traditional spaces may also be used to showcase artwork and to reach diverse audiences; examples are the Institute of Mental Health in Nottingham, UK (see Case Study 6.2; Institute of Mental Health, 2014) and disused shops which reach large numbers of people including those who may never enter a gallery or museum.

Case Study 6.2 *Art beyond the gallery: showing work in non-traditional spaces*

Since 2009 the Institute of Mental Health in Nottingham, UK has displayed artwork by people with mental health problems. The author VT was appointed arts coordinator for the Institute and has overseen a range of creative activities, 'Art at the Institute', encompassing exhibition, education and curation (see www.institutemh.org.uk/x-about-us-x/art-at-the-institute). Crucially the Institute is a working office building housing around 200 staff who work on clinical, educational and research programmes aiming to improve the lives of people with mental health problems. The building is visited by thousands of people each year attending training, meetings and events. Beginning with just a handful of donated and purchased artworks, there is now a rolling programme of exhibitions on themes like 'voices', 'identity' and 'recovery'. Many different issues have been depicted artistically including self-harm, depression, medication, suicidal ideation, attention deficit hyperactivity disorder and seasonal affective disorder.

The exhibitions have enabled over 200 artists from all over the UK to show their work, all of whom are invited to the Institute to see the work on display and to talk to staff and visitors about it. Many of these artists are untrained and for those who have formal training it is often the first time they have displayed work in a non-traditional space. Artists may sell their work if they choose to, providing a source of income for those on low incomes and signifying a change in status from patient to artist. The exhibitions provide a stimulating work environment for staff and visitors, and create an open environment in which discussion about personal experiences of mental illness are encouraged. The exhibitions have an impact on the artists who may feel marginalised and stigmatised due to their illness and experiences of mental health care. Some displays have proved controversial, for example art shown posthumously – produced by an individual who had committed suicide (see Tischler, in press) – and work on religious themes. This has stimulated consultation and debate engaging a wide range of individuals, thus demonstrating the potential of art to shift and shape attitudes. 'Art at the Institute' demonstrates that non-traditional environments can be successfully utilised to provide space for individuals to display their artwork, particularly those who would have limited or no similar opportunities, to expose individuals to work that stimulates discussion about mental illness and mental health care, and to reach a wider audience than may visit an art gallery.

What's the Evidence?

Many of the studies focusing on artistic engagement have methodological limitations. Systematic or realist reviews of visual art interventions indicate that often analysis and outcomes are poorly described (e.g. Beard, 2011) and use of arts-based methods in research is often criticised for lacking theoretical context (Fraser and al Sayah, 2011). Most research to date has tended to focus on participatory engagement rather than receptive perception of visual art in healthcare (Moss et al., 2012). Additionally there are debates about what constitutes evidence in this field. For example, some argue that the benefits of engagement with art are so obvious so as to make empirical investigation unnecessary. Others suggest that the visual arts should be subject to scrutiny as with any such approach utilised therapeutically, especially if it is being recommended as part of a healthcare regime. Particular aspects such as health economic benefits remain to be fully explored in visual arts interventions. From a pragmatic perspective an intervention that is offered within a health or social care context and is funded by the taxpayer ought to demonstrate its effectiveness. Yet the issue of what constitutes evidence remains a lively interdisciplinary topic of debate. In particular, issues of process and experience are difficult to assess using standardised measurements and work is ongoing to develop novel methodologies that may fully represent these types of interventions, such as visual and documentary systems (e.g. Reavey, 2011).

Engaging the Public

Visual art represents a powerful tool for public engagement with healthcare research. There is now increased emphasis on translating research for public consumption and making research data relevant and engaging. This provides opportunities for visual art to showcase and interpret work which may be complex and dense in scientific detail. The phenomenon of the peak shift is relevant here as work can be distilled and developed, providing an educational function whilst allowing the artist scope to produce something novel. Work at the interface of science and art, the so-called 'sciart' field, is gaining prominence, with organisations such as the Wellcome Trust in London, UK (see www.wellcome.ac.uk) pioneering collaboration between the arts and healthcare. Their exhibitions explore a wide range of conditions and issues relevant to healthcare including mental illness, addiction, sex neuroscience, the history of anatomical knowledge, and death and dying. Such exhibitions reveal the potential of art to both educate and arouse aesthetic responses.

Exhibitions may also educate as well as showcase and interpret research on healthcare themes, for example in the area of mental health. The 'Art in the Asylum' exhibition at the Djanogly Gallery, Nottingham, UK in 2013 focused on the history of mental health care, the therapeutic and diagnostic use of art within asylums, and the reception of patient art into the wider cultural scene – for

Case Study 6.3 *Art in the Asylum*

A major international exhibition, 'Art in the Asylum: Creativity and the Evolution of Psychiatry', charting the use of artistic activity in British asylums, was held in the UK in 2013. The exhibition focused on the diagnostic and therapeutic use of art in asylums dating from the 19th century, and also explored the reception by the art world of work created by people with mental health problems.

Whist the exhibition aimed to visually explore medico-historical perspectives, it was equally a vehicle for educating a diverse range of visitors about mental health and the care of those experiencing mental illness. A wide range of educational and learning programmes were held alongside the exhibition in the form of talks, workshops and panel discussions. These engaged a variety of attendees and encouraged discussion and debate about mental health issues such as cognitive behavioural therapy, electro-convulsive therapy and hospitalisation. Thousands of people visited the exhibition and associated events including groups of schoolchildren, and students from disciplines such as art therapy, nursing, medicine, fine art and counselling. This highlights the value of open-access community venues and visual stimuli to engage a wide range of people with health issues.

example by artists from the Surrealist movement – and aimed to stimulate the interest of the public at the same time as disseminating important and useful information about healthcare (see Case Study 6.3). Accessible, public events such as these create a climate of openness, encourage participation and debate, and challenge stigma associated with illness.

Moving Beyond Boundaries: Realising the Potential of Visual Art in Health in the Future

This chapter has highlighted the current and potential contributions of the visual arts to enhancing human health individually and collectively, through therapy, education and exhibition. Further interdisciplinary collaboration is essential to effectively extend the role of art in healthcare and to develop work which is effective and theoretically progressive. This involves artists, art therapists and art historians working with those from disciplines such as medicine, nursing and psychology. Such interdisciplinary working is gaining momentum and is often a requirement of research bids. Although this style of working is highly stimulating and creative, it is also challenging. Sharing and learning across different philosophical, theoretical and practical paradigms is not easy, yet recent work indicates that this area is where novel and groundbreaking developments lie.

Structural issues are also prevalent. There remains a chasm between the humanities and the sciences with ongoing debates regarding the nature of 'evidence', and biomedical science is still the most dominant and powerful lobby within health research and practice. Increased interdisciplinary work in this field is beginning to erode these boundaries, yet more needs to be done to exploit the full potential of the arts to benefit health. Networks beyond delivery which address the interface of interdisciplinarity and the unique possibilities for advanced learning and theory are to be commended.

Summary and Conclusions

This chapter has identified key areas in which visual art is making an impact in health research, education and provision. Although art is being utilised to process individual experiences of illness, to facilitate personal and research communication in a wider societal context, and to enhance clinical and non-clinical environments, there is scope for a much greater role for visual art within health humanities and beyond. Art represents a cultural, aesthetic and historical mode of representation, one which is immediately potent due to the dominance of our visual sense and the visual culture in which we exist, and as such can be a catalyst to enhance health and well-being.

7
Practice Based Evidence: Delivering Humanities into Healthcare

The title of this chapter could imply several things. First, it could cover the way evidence is derived from practice. Certainly, we will consider this later as this process is uniquely suited to the kinds of humanities interventions which are applied in healthcare contexts. Second, it could cover the kinds of evidence that may be needed in order to place humanities-based activities on the healthcare agenda and drive their inclusion in healthcare practice. Yes, this too will be among our considerations. But the relationship between the humanities, the idea of evidence and healthcare itself, is a lot more complicated than that. There are different cultures of what counts as evidence, conflicting ideas about how best to conduct human inquiry and tensions between the world of research and the world of practitioners. Therefore in this chapter one of our central tasks will be to explore what these cultures are and how they have evolved along different trajectories, as well as offering some ideas for their rapprochement to the benefit of scholars and practitioners as well as patients and informal carers.

Perhaps the best way to start is to consider the idea of evidence based practice. This has been an underlying principle of healthcare in many parts of the world for a generation now and has driven a whole range of debates about how best to evaluate healthcare interventions, how to fund research and how to educate and develop practitioners and researchers. It is with these powerful notions of evidence based practice and evidence based medicine that alternative ideas have had to compete to be taken seriously.

120

Therefore an appropriate way to begin our story is with the concept of evidence based practice itself, before we consider what its alternative – practice based evidence – might look like. This will enable us to consider the final part of the title, namely how best humanities interventions might be promoted and delivered in sometimes conservative healthcare environments and organisations.

An early definition of evidence based practice by Sackett et al. (1996, p. 71) still commands considerable assent amongst practitioners and researchers. It is 'the conscientious, explicit and judicious use of current best evidence in making decisions about the care of individual patients, based on the skills which allow the doctor (sic) to evaluate both personal experience and external evidence in a systematic and objective manner'.

In evidence based practice, a hierarchy of evidence tends to be set up, ranging from the highly trustworthy through to the least certain. This hierarchy, which is apt to be promoted on both sides of the Atlantic, tends to place randomised controlled trials – experiments, in other words – at the top of the list. Here, for example, is the kind of typology of evidence presented by the UK's Department of Health (1996). In descending order of credibility it includes:

I. Strong evidence from at least one systematic review of multiple well-designed randomised controlled trials.
II. Strong evidence from at least one properly designed randomised controlled trial of appropriate size.
III. Evidence from well-designed trials such as non-randomised trials, cohort studies, time series or matched case-controlled studies.
IV. Evidence from well-designed non-experimental studies from more than one centre or research group.
V. Opinions of respected authorities, based on clinical evidence, descriptive studies or reports of expert committees.

Thus, in this view the only thing better than a randomised controlled trial is a large number of these which are so similar that their data (or perhaps some statistical measure of effect size) can be added together in a meta-analysis or systematic review. This then is the evidence on which practitioners are encouraged to base their work.

As we have noted elsewhere (Brown et al., 2003), the arguments in favour of evidence based practice are commonsensically persuasive on scientific, humanitarian and politico-economic grounds. The spectacle of expensive and ineffective interventions falling to the astute gaze of perspicacious researchers is an attractive one. In principle, it seems to be endorsed as a service philosophy amongst many healthcare staff.

The dominance of the large scale randomised controlled clinical trial as a way of finding out what works in healthcare has been challenged on a number of counts. For example, as Warner and Spandler (2012) point out, smaller scale, qualitative studies may be better to meet the everyday concerns of service providers and users. However, given the minatory power of hierarchies like Sackett et al.'s, research like this tends to carry less weight in the development of health policy and clinical guidelines. In the UK, bodies such as the Cochrane Collaboration and the National Institute of Clinical Excellence attempt to direct practice in terms of the highly valued evidence. There are, therefore, significant tensions among policymakers, practitioners and service users as far as the merits of different types of 'evidence' are concerned.

'But it's a bit more complicated': Limitations of the Evidence Based Practice Model

The traditional view, that the best scientific evidence should inform practice, is what Bracken (2007) has called the 'technological paradigm'. This is dominant in a variety of fields, including healthcare and especially in mental health. Put crudely, the 'technological paradigm' assumes that we can identify a set of interventions and study them as they are applied to particular patient groups. Moreover, it is assumed that we can study them relatively independently of context, relationships and values. It is as if we were able to say 'here's a storytelling initiative for people with postnatal depression', 'here's a visual arts intervention with nursing students', or 'here's an art therapy group for people with schizophrenia' and so on. Now let's see if people who've been through this intervention are doing any better than similar people who haven't. That looks sensible enough at first glance. But let us unpack some of the stages in this process. First of all, it's hard to cleanly define groups of people like this. Especially in mental health, grouping people on the basis of symptoms or diagnoses may not make much sense as the boundaries between categories and the way in which people are assigned to them are often ambiguous (Kinghorn, 2011; Whooley, 2010). In addition, people often have complex multiple health problems and needs. Disorders (if we can call them that) rarely occur in isolation and often show high degrees of co-morbidity such that people may have multiple mental and physical health problems at once (Cunningham et al., 2013) and may relate to a whole range of other psychosocial aspects of the situation like coping resources, physical activity and social relationships (Di Benedetto et al., 2014). So in practice it is often difficult to be precise about what is wrong with people and what exactly it is that the intervention is addressing.

Let us suppose, however, that we can define a group of people for whom an intervention works. For example, if we found that poetry therapy improves resilience and reduces anxiety in people with cancer, as Tegner et al. (2009) did, does this mean that it's a good thing to roll out to everyone with cancer? Well, most people reading this would feel that it is a good idea at a personal level, but let us consider the reasoning process behind this. It would involve grouping people together on the basis of their diagnosis as 'cancer patients' and offering them interventions that seem to have the best results for the majority – the 'best average'. As a number of authors point out (Bola and Mosher, 2002; Warner and Spandler, 2012) this often comes about at the expense of individualised, flexible and tailor made support. As we have suggested above, the similarity of clients on the basis of a diagnostic category may be uncertain. In Warner and Spandler's case they remark that lumping together people who self-injure and people who make suicide attempts is often done, but may be problematic. In addition, the suitability of, and patients' response to, an intervention may be contoured by a variety of wider social inequalities related to social class, age, gender, sexuality and ethnicity, although these are often strongly correlated with long-term health problems (Rogers and Pilgrim, 2003).

Practice Based Evidence: Doing Justice to the Richness of Practice

To foreground the alternate view, that much can be learned in practice itself, a number of authors have proposed a countervailing concept, that of 'practice based evidence', which is said to offer a bottom-up means of gathering evidence from the experience of everyday practice, drawing on the expertise of practitioners and service users to inform recommendations for future practice and, ultimately, policy (Lucock et al., 2003; Margison et al., 2000; Warner and Spandler, 2012).

Warner and Spandler (2012) argue that research should try to incorporate service users' own values and aspirations and thereby provide more holistic and contextual understandings of clinical practice. The focus on meaning which they advocate tends more often to be found in qualitative approaches to research. Accordingly, Warner and Spandler propose that we should conceptualise research so as to combine aspects which include cognitive, emotional *and* more nuanced behavioural data. In this way, they say, research can elicit information which is meaningful to practitioners and service users and produce evidence which is also robust enough for policymakers and those who commission services.

This chimes in with a feeling on the part of many practitioners in a variety of healthcare disciplines that there is more to what goes on in their work than what evidence based practice can capture. Meanings, feelings, culture, dreams, relationships and reflections are often hard to apprehend via the medium of randomised controlled trials. Consequently, there are for example pleas for the rubric of nursing to extend beyond evidence based practice to include information literacy, the humanities, ethics and the social sciences (Jutel, 2008). Especially in mental health nursing, the arts have often been employed as diversional and therapeutic interventions, and for both therapy and education – as we quoted earlier, 'art offers a showing of human experience in unique ways' (Biley and Galvin, 2007, p. 806) to promote and enact shared understanding of people's experiences. Many of these issues can only be crudely characterised in ways which would make sense within a clinical trial. It is often not an easy task to unpack what is happening within an arts or humanities intervention and in what way it has most impact.

There are similar problems with the idea of practice based evidence. As Fox (2003) points out, there is a great deal of social science research into 'practice', in healthcare as well as a variety of other fields – social services, education, youth work and so on – which provides a great deal of data on how services are delivered. In some cases this provides valuable recommendations for improving services.

However, very often academic researchers do not take the time to push these ideas through into practice. It is as if research has ended as soon as the report is written to the funders, the paper has been accepted for publication, seminars have been given and participants and stakeholders have all gone home.

Wood et al. (1998) found that practitioners felt that disembodied research findings were not convincing, but wanted instead to see these findings contextualised in terms of their own professional experience. Wood et al. argued that in order for adoption to occur it was necessary that practitioners 'bought in' to the proposed changes, and for research to take into account locally-situated practices through which practitioners engage with the research. 'Research findings' do not necessarily represent 'truth' about reality, as one 'reified moment' in the ongoing saga of 'practice' (Wood et al., 1998, p. 1735).

The Question of Evidence and the Humanities: Difficulties of Evaluation Perspective and the Politics of Knowledge

In terms of unfolding an evidence based rationale for humanities interventions, this too is fraught with difficulty when we consider what humanities-based interventions and their originators say about themselves. This is relatively rarely phrased in terms of outcome measures and key performance indicators. To take an example, let us look at how we might conceptualise the effects of an intervention based on fairy tales or folktales (Sommer et al., 2012). Folklorist Maria Tatar (1999) has explored what she sees to be the value of fairy tales at both individual and community levels. She notes 'their widespread and enduring popularity' and claims that they perform 'a significant social function...' (p. xi). She continues that our enduring fascination in stories like these is part of a desire 'to develop maps' to enable people to cope with complex personal, familial and social frustrations encountered in everyday life (p. xi). A fellow folklorist, Jack Zipes (2006) of the University of Minnesota, propounds the idea that fairy tales are a 'metaphorical mode of communication' which people use to understand both themselves and the social world around them (p. 95). These kinds of claims are not unusual amongst students of folklore and fairy tales. The difficulty in formally evaluating these assertions is not particularly crucial since their truth lies in their persuasiveness and their ability to generate insightful ways of looking at folklore – what function is it performing for the people concerned and what sense do they make of it? The question of how we might evaluate these sorts of claims and what we might do about testing them becomes more critical when we consider the growing popularity of narratives and stories in psychotherapy and counselling. As a narrative counsellor, Barclay (2007) also indicated that stories serve a similar function. He noted that 'in the context of cultural myths, stories soothe people with the analogies that they provide, normalizing, through metaphor, the vicissitudes of life's travails' (p. 1). Brown and Augusta-Scott (2007) propose that stories and their re-telling serve an epistemological function – that is, they are concerned with the nature of knowledge. In their view, it is more or less impossible to know the world directly – indeed this is fundamental to the approach as much narrative psychotherapy adopts a social constructionist view of the world. Instead we turn to 'lived experiences' and alternative stories or 'alternative story possibilities' (p. xii). Indeed, Speedy (2000) suggests that work with stories 'would acknowledge the multi-storied possibilities available' (p. 419). And Tatar (1999) notes that where stories are concerned, 'few fairy tales dictate a single, univocal, uncontested meaning; most are so elastic as to accommodate a wide variety of interpretations, and they derive their meaning through a process of engaged negotiation on the part of the reader' (p. xiv). Thus stories offer multiple opportunities for individual interpretations which can allow clients (and maybe practitioners too) to examine their own difficulties through this process of mutually negotiated meaning.

Scientific research in the era of post-Enlightenment modernity, and the kind of work which is highly valued in the evidence based practice movement, has this kind of search for truth as its goal. Through observation and reasoning and progressive refinement of theory, knowledge will approximate ever more closely to 'truth' (Popper, 1982). In this framework, the aim of research is to observe, analyse and understand aspects of the world in causal, material terms. Consequently, the mutual negotiation of meaning and the analysis of experience which we have described here are unlikely to satisfy the requirements of a form of inquiry that demands the evaluation of knowledge claims in this way. Moreover, as the academy has evolved in the latter part of the 20th century a variety of other voices have demanded that peoples, groups and kinds of experience that have hitherto been marginalised should be heard.

For example, Ramazanoglu has argued (1992, p. 209) that a specifically feminist approach to methodology has arisen as a result of power struggles over what it means to 'know' and what counts as valid research. The feminist commitment to resisting patriarchy has been accompanied by a suspicion of grand narratives (Holmwood, 1995, p. 416) and instead entertains a preference for research which is local, engaged with women's concerns and which values experience (Gelsthorpe, 1992, p. 214; Oakley, 1998, p. 708).

Within feminism, as with other critical forms of inquiry, many writers have drawn attention to the differences in power between the researcher and the researched. Research often involves relatively privileged people looking at those who are more marginalised. The participants in research are often those whose gender, ethnicity or sexuality places them in a marginalised or minority position. Alternatively, their status as patients, offenders, clients of social services, or pupils in schools means that they are disadvantaged in terms of expertise and social power. Other writers have explored the relationship between the person doing the research and the person on whom the research is being done from a variety of theoretical perspectives.

Research has often involved those who are in powerful positions eliciting information from and scrutinising those with less power. Elite groups do research on people in poverty, criminologists do research on offenders, and doctors and medical researchers corral patients into clinical trials. Elite groups themselves – senior managers, politicians and the like – are often far less intensively investigated and have more control over how they are presented. These power relationships in research have been a focus of concern especially for feminist scholars. Landmark publications in this area include Stanley and Wise (1983) and their feminist exposé of power relationships in research or Oakley's (e.g. 1991) ground breaking studies of childbirth in which she examined the role of relationships in research and the way that rather than simply discovering new truths about the human condition this was often a two-way transaction in which the women in the study had many questions for the researcher.

In the 1990s there was a good deal of interest in the potential of postmodernism in the social sciences to open up opportunities for hitherto marginalised voices to be heard. Moreover, there were attempts to problematise the roles of the actors involved. For example, Stronach and MacLure (1997) argued that the concept of a 'researcher' is a construction achieved in opposition to definitions of practitioner or a research participant (1997, p. 100).

Practice Based Research: New Approaches, New Validities

In the 1990s spirit of postmodernism a number of authors argued for new approaches to make sense of the research process. Rather than the well-worn notion of validity (whether you are measuring what you think you're measuring) there was some discussion of a novel construct, that of 'transgressive validity' in research, as outlined by Lather (1993, p. 676; DeLuca, 2011). In this view, the 'validity' of research is to do with its ability to transgress, challenge or subvert existing conceptions of the topic area. Lather's application of transgressive validity to social science research sought to de-centre traditional ideas and 'reframe validity as multiple, partial, endlessly deferred' (1993, p. 675). In this conception of the human inquiry process the transgressive mode of working fundamentally problematises the traditional ideas of truth derived from positivism and instead seeks to reconceptualise 'the very criteria of validity' through critical questioning of culturally biased assumptions (Moss, 1996, p. 26).

In this way, says Fox (2003), we can imagine and implement 'practice-oriented research that is constitutive of difference, challenges power and constraint and encourages resistance and new possibilities' (p. 89). Among a number of newer approaches to thinking about research, the idea of transgressive validity is helpful in prompting a critical stance towards validity, evidence and validity criteria. In a similar vein, as Ledwith (2007) says of emancipatory action research, there is more to the business of being critical than simply enabling participation. Whilst it is valuable for researchers to enable meaningful participation on the part of the people they are researching, and promote collaboration, a more fully emancipatory approach goes a step further than simple participatory research and may involve the participants in the research helping to define problems, identify research questions and implement research activities, as well as trying to find ways of using the research to bring about social change. In this way, research aims to be empowering and transformatory. For example, White and Robson's (2011) account of work in arts and health in schools in the north-east of England describes how sustained programmes of participatory arts activity and shared creativity can contribute to bottom-up expressions of public health. They can at the same time help identify and address the specific local health needs of a community. This kind of action work, involving creative activity, research and ambitions towards effective social change, combines personal experience and facilitating people's engagement with their own health needs, and also creates 'commitment to a communal will for a shared experience' (White and Robson, 2011, p. 54).

This species of activity, integrating action and intervention with research and an agenda for change, may well rely at a basic level on dialogue, dialectic, interpretive and hermeneutic modes of inquiry which may yield very different ideas about reality depending on whose perspective is considered. Indeed, as veteran action researcher Michelle Fine (e.g. Stoudt et al., 2012) has frequently argued, objectivity may well turn out to be not so much about truth, but to represent the standpoint of a dominant group. Hence, democratising methods and involving people in helping to define reality can itself serve to provide interpretive evidence for validity arguments themselves. Indeed, in examining the role of the creative arts in humane medicine, McLean (2014) highlights how people who have often not had a voice in the past can be surprised that practitioners and researchers are suddenly taking an interest in their point of view.

A further example of how participation and practice can change the agenda, perspective and debates comes from Matarasso (2012), who examines the role of the arts in older adults and the part they might play in successful ageing. Art among the elderly can be considerably more than the pleasant diversion it is usually thought to be. It can be a fundamental means of negotiating one's place and purpose in society. In Matarasso's work there is hardly any mention of the usual agenda of infirmity and disability but rather a focus on creative engagement and flourishing. Indeed, it is only in retirement that some of Matarasso's informants had finally been able to fulfil long-cherished creative ambitions.

The commitment to changing the terms of debate or changing the world is one facet of the notion of transgressive validity we mentioned earlier. Much of what one might do in this variety of research owes a good deal of its shape and form to the principles of 'emancipatory' action research outlined by Carr and Kemmis (1986) nearly 30 years ago. However, the idea of transgressive validity foregrounds a principle of difference rather than convergence on a shared rationality. As originally conceived, the idea of transgressive research is a reflexive one. As Stronach and MacLure (1997) comment, in the spirit of transgressive validity, this concept itself would necessarily be subject to transgression.

Despite this awareness of reflexive possibilities, the transgressive spirit in research does not necessarily lead to stasis or navel gazing. The concept of 'transgressive research' and the transgressive approach attempt to interrogate the evidence for hegemonic imbalances in order to discover the political underpinnings of experience and practice. For example, Furman (2006) discusses the role of poetry in exploring the experience of illness and hospitalisation. As he says:

> Successful expressive poems are based on empirical data that are sensory and evocative in nature. Imagistic language allows the reader to enter a work and develop his or her own personal relationship with it; the images are transformed into knowledge pertaining to both the poem and the reader. (Furman, 2006, p. 561)

Furman's poems relate to a period of hospitalisation with troubling symptoms of respiratory distress and imagistically and evocatively record the sights and sounds, anticipation of one's own death and interaction with staff and loved ones. Moreover, as the poetry evolves it comes to resonate with other much earlier forms of poetic storytelling from different cultures such as the so-called 'tanka' or the repetitive 'pantoum' form.

In the case of Furman's work, the aim is to use poetic forms to produce something meaningful but in a way which runs counter 'to the standard validity of correspondence: a non-referential validity interested in how discourse does its work' (Lather, 1993, p. 675). In presenting experiences poetically this kind of approach recalls the famous social scientist Norman Denzin's (1997) advocacy of using alternative forms of data in order to evoke deep and compelling emotional responses on the part of the reader of research. Accordingly, the expressive and creative arts have the potential to expand understanding, represent in new ways subtle ideas or notions that might be paradoxical or dialectic, and lend themselves to the conceptualisation of experiences and processes that are difficult to reduce.

Following the implications of this for our discussion of how research might be understood and evaluated, let us return briefly to Lather (1993) and DeLuca (2011) who outline some lesser appreciated but nonetheless useful aspects of the idea of validity which may be especially useful when the arts and humanities in health are under scrutiny:

1. The first of these validities is what Lather calls simulacra/ironic validity, which involves raising questions about the representation of validity. In this view the notion of truth itself is something that should be problematised. All validity evidence is at least one step removed from real experience, and through our language, which is always an incomplete and partial representation of reality, experience is placed in symbolic form which may therefore be communicable, but is somewhat different from what gave rise to it.

2. The second form of transgressive validity which Lather identifies is what she calls the paralogical form of validity, in which the need for logical resolution is avoided and the opportunity for incommensurable forms of evidence is allowed. This form of validity reminds us to resist the urge to clean up nature and resolve incongruent evidences from validity arguments. Here, the aim also is to embody 'a situated, partial, positioned, explicit tentativeness' (Lather, 1993, p. 685).

3. Thirdly, Lather considers rhizomatic validity. The idea of a rhizome in philosophy and the social sciences is borrowed from Deleuze and Guattari (1980) and describes theory and research that allow for multiple, non-hierarchical entry and exit points in data representation and interpretation. This they distinguish from the conventional tree like 'arborescent' representation of knowledge which charts causality along chronological lines and looks for the original source of 'things' and looks towards their pinnacle or conclusion. A rhizome on the other hand is concerned with ongoing connections between chains of meaning, organisations of power, and circumstances relative to the arts, sciences and social struggles.

4. Fourthly and finally, Lather's voluptuous validity encourages us to seek out ethics through practices of engagement and self-reflexivity (Lather, 1993, pp. 685–686). This kind of approach has often been identified with a feminine principle as distinct from the masculine principle of 'hard' data. It concerns the extent and nature of the researcher's engagement with the participants and their sensual world. Indeed, the enjoyment of things like music, drama, poetry or the visual arts are sensory, and often sensual, experiences. Under the heading of voluptuous validity we might also examine how validation practices and theories typically reflect a more powerful male perspective. Further, voluptuous validity reminds us of the need to examine validity processes and the kinds of evidence that relate to these from multiple perspectives including those of diverse genders, cultures and political positions.

Going back to our original concern about the nature of evidence in the health humanities and the kinds of ways in which evidence might inform and also be derived from practice, we hope it has become clear that this is not a simple issue. The reliance of much discourse about evidence based practice on randomised controlled trials places many of the interventions in the arts and humanities at a disadvantage because they are often not evaluated in this way, and unlike drug treatment, it is difficult to imagine an adequate placebo which could be given instead of the active treatment. On the other hand, there is the possibility of practice based evidence. This is a rich field and, as we have demonstrated in this volume, there is a wealth of experience. Yet thinking about the experience of practitioners, researchers and participants in practice is by no means straightforward. As feminist and postmodernist scholars have pointed out, whose reality we privilege and how we turn experience into research reports is fraught with difficulty. Practice – at least if it is performed sensitively and thoughtfully – does not yield a single reality that can be turned into 'evidence'.

As a consequence, a good deal of what we learn about the role of the arts and humanities in health is in the form of knowledges that cleave most readily to interpretive, narrative or postmodern styles of inquiry. There are a great many precedents for trying to make sense of this – from feminism, postmodernism itself and a variety of hermeneutic and interpretive styles of work. Thus any single analysis can only be presented as a 'tentative statement opening upon a limitless field of possible interpretations' (Churchill, 2000, p. 164). Savin-Baden and Fisher (2002) write of allowing researchers to 'acknowledge that trust and truth are fragile' while enabling them 'to engage with the messiness and complexity of data interpretation in ways that ... reflect the lives of ... participants' (p. 191). Now, most texts about research methods would claim that it is not appropriate to generalise or extrapolate findings from qualitative studies. However, this need not be seen as a blanket prohibition. Rather it is a call to modesty and tentativeness in our findings. As Kersten et al. (2010) propose, if we are sufficiently explicit about the circumstances of the study, the recruitment of participants, the methods used and the researcher's role, readers will be able to judge how relevant the knowledge in question is to their own (Sandelowski et al., 1997). Indeed, in some cases research and writing in the health humanities may yield 'knowledge claims that are so powerful and convincing in their own right they ... carry the validation with them, like a strong piece of art' (Kvale, 1996, p. 252).

Evaluating Research: How Do We Know It Will Work?

Martyn Hammersley (1992), in a volume entitled *What's Wrong with Ethnography?*, proposed that ethnographic work should be evaluated in terms of its *plausibility and credibility* – that is, are there sufficient data presented to support the credibility of the findings? Hammersley also proposes that we should consider the relevance of the study in the sense of offering valuable new information on the topic or making a contribution to the literature. He also notes the importance of the audience to which the account of research is addressed. What will be needed for a medical journal will differ from what might work in a presentation to an informal carers' group, for example.

There are many further contributions to the debate on how we can evaluate qualitative research. Finlay (2007) talks about clarity (does it make sense?), credibility (is it convincing?), contribution (is it adding to our knowledge?) and communicative resonance (does it draw readers in?). Madill et al. (2000) offer the notions of *internal coherence*, *deviant case analysis* and *reader evaluation*. By internal coherence they mean the extent to which a given analysis 'hangs together' logically without contradictions. Deviant case analysis involves considering outliers and data that do not appear to fit the analytic scheme. Reader evaluation relates to the extent to which the study yields insight and understanding for the reader. Madill et al. recommend that we rely extensively on verbatim quotations from the data to enable readers to derive their own interpretations. As they go on, 'qualitative researchers have a responsibility to make their epistemological position clear, conduct their research in a manner consistent with that position, and present their findings in a way that allows them to be evaluated properly' (Madill et al., 2000, p. 17).

As the stock of knowledge about health humanities interventions grows, we need to consider how it might be possible to aggregate or compile the various studies or strands of information. In the last few years the technique of metasynthesis has been proposed as a means of bringing the diversity of qualitative research together. Rather like its cousins systematic review and meta-analysis, this initially involves identifying appropriate terms with which to search the available literature, but the mode of analysis is thematic rather than statistical.

Noblit and Hare (1988) suggest that there are three stages to conducting a metasynthesis:

1. The reciprocal stage – recognising recurring themes and ideas where the reviewer identifies what these recurrent themes are, which sources they are in and how often they occur.
2. The refutational stage – recognising themes and ideas that go against the common themes and ideas.
3. The line of argument – constructing a statement that can summarise and express what has been found.

For example, a metasynthesis examining studies of the experiences of living after a stroke found remarkably similar findings in the nine sources included (Salter et al., 2008). Salter et al.'s metasynthesis suggested firstly a sudden, overwhelming and fundamental life change for the stroke survivor. There is also a widely reported sense of loss, uncertainty and social isolation in conjunction with the process of transition and transformation. However, a further theme concerns the capability of the survivor for adaptation and reconciliation of identity, enabling them to move forward towards meaningful recovery.

In addition, the kinds of interpretive inquiries which take place in the health humanities may increasingly find themselves occurring in conjunction with other methods in complex evaluative programmes of research. The popularity of mixed methods approaches to evaluate complex interventions is growing, with many funding bodies (e.g. the UK Medical Research Council, 2008) recommending that randomised controlled trials should be supplemented by qualitative research. In connection with this, Daly et al. (2007) suggest a hierarchy for judging the value of qualitative research as a basis for action for practitioners or policy. Daly et al. would attach more weight to conceptually sophisticated studies that analyse all available data according to conceptual themes. Even so, there may be limitations as a result of a lack of diversity in the sample. More readily generalisable studies, they say, will be ones which use conceptual frameworks to derive an appropriately diversified sample as well as attempting to account for all data. The least likely studies to produce convincing, practically relevant evidence are single case studies. A study which is largely descriptive may provide interesting lists of quotations but in the absence of detailed conceptual analysis it may have little to contribute to the broader field of practice.

Daly et al. (2007) also contend that qualitative studies may have a variety of uses such as illuminating treatment issues – for instance exploring why some clients respond better to some interventions – and in formulating critique of current practice. It is often through detailed qualitative analysis that we become aware that standard practice may not be benefitting one or more groups of people. In the broader health field qualitative analysis may help us identify the variables and factors which may be critical in providing evidence for or against interventions and programmes and lay the foundations for evidence relevant to the creation of better health policy.

Summary and Conclusions

Finally, do we always need randomised controlled trials before we can deliver a humanities-based activity in healthcare? Surely the answer here is 'no' for the reasons we have described earlier. Do we need to question and interrogate the evidence for what we do? The answer to this is undeniably 'yes'. Surely we will need some assurance that what we do will be better than doing nothing, and we will often need to demonstrate this to those who have their hands on the purse strings. The best answers about how to improve outcomes for patients will very likely arise from integrating a variety of suitable methods (Upshur et al., 2001). It is vital that different kinds of knowledge are valued, understood and most importantly integrated if we, as service users, investigators, practitioners or commissioners, are to reach towards a more complete picture of what may be going on when the humanities are applied in healthcare.

8
Creative Practice as Mutual Recovery

There is a clear opportunity for the emergent field of health humanities to move to a whole new level of impact, with contributions from anthropology, narrative and literature to linguistics, music and visual art, as well as the very many arts and humanities-based knowledges and practices that it was not possible to include in this slim manifesto volume. As we have indicated, creative practice is a major activity in societies worldwide, and arts and expressive therapies are well established in physical and mental health services. In terms of the latter, for example, research has already demonstrated the importance of arts for 'recovery orientated mental health services' (Spandler et al., 2007), how they provide ways of breaking down social barriers, of expressing and understanding experiences and emotions, and of helping to rebuild identities and communities (Brown and Kandirikirira, 2007; Devlin, 2009; Secker et al., 2007).

The creative practices in both the arts and humanities are set to become a mainstream mechanism for social connectedness and recovery for all involved in healthcare, that is, the healthcare workforce alongside patients and informal carers. Arguably, what is coming down the track is more radical and transformative than what has been achieved to date under a 'therapy' umbrella. Creative practice has documented potential for having a unique role to play not just in advancing mutual recovery but also in transforming future approaches to non-professional solutions for physical and mental health and well-being. The notion of 'mutual recovery' (Crawford et al., 2013b) was seeded many years ago when author

PC found himself working in a less than ideal mental hospital with an environment of decline and reduced resources for the recovery of its patients.

PC's Encounter with Mutual Recovery

The professionals were doing their best but in a dispiriting climate. I felt the gravity of this poor environment and found myself struggling to maintain a positive mentality. 'How the hell did I end up here?' I asked myself as if I were on a section of the Mental Health Act and not one of our more disturbed patients. It was depressing and I began to wonder whether working in healthcare, and mental health in particular, was the best thing for my own health and well-being. I questioned where the emotional and intellectual energy to care for patients would come from. How could I add to their lives when my own seemed so compromised? Then, one day, I was walking along the hospital's filthy main corridor and heard music. It was simply beautiful and I went in search of the source. Half-expecting to come across someone with a radio or music player, I found instead, one of the patients sitting on the floor outside his ward, playing a clarinet. It was no ordinary performance. It was raw, lyrical and stunning. The impact of the music on me was clear. I stopped and soaked it up. My tense shoulders unfolded, my breathing stilled, my face relaxed and my eyes closed in reverent reception. My mouth curled gently upwards, my body lifted and I remember the slow inhalation of a different air through my nose as if taking the music deep inside by this route as well as my ears. At that moment, although not conscious of this at the time, I was being recovered. It was not me recovering the needy patient. It was the patient-musician recovering me. It is here that I began to consider who is recovering whom? I learned later that the man playing the clarinet was one of the UK's most revered jazz musicians.

The issue of who is recovering whom is radically important because, if we were to listen only to traditional medical perspectives on mental health, and healthcare in general, one would be hard pressed to see the patient as anything other than recipient of professional care and the professional carer or therapist as the sole agent of recovery for the patient. But should we continue in this mode? Should we only view the professional carer or therapist as contributor and solution provider to those with health challenges? Conversely, should we only view patients and informal carers as drawing from professional expertise and not offering back social and cultural capital that restores and underpins formal caregivers and therapists, thus enhancing communities of care? After all, informal carers, health and social care staff, and even education staff with well-being agendas, for example, are subject to high stress, mental health problems and burnout (Edwards et al., 2000; Pinquart and Sörensen, 2003; Rudow, 1999) and need recovering. It is our view that we need a major paradigm shift in this regard.

In a highly collaborative major study funded by the Arts and Humanities Research Council/Research Councils UK, currently underway and outlined in Crawford et al. (2013b), we have been seeking to examine how creative practice in the arts and humanities can promote the kinds of connectedness and reciprocity that support 'mutual recovery' in terms of mental health and well-being. But there is no reason to assume that this idea should be limited to mental health. It is equally pertinent to general healthcare and public health provision.

The idea of 'mutual recovery' extends out of the increasingly influential notion of 'recovery' in mental health care which refers to the possibility of achieving a meaningful and more resilient life irrespective of mental health 'symptoms' or disabilities. Typically, however, recovery-based initiatives tend to focus exclusively on people identified as having health needs (service users) and overlook how hard-pressed informal carers and health, social care and education personnel may also need to 'recover' or be 'recovered' in terms of their own general/mental health and well-being. In other words, the central hypothesis here is that creative practice could be a powerful tool for bringing together a range of social actors and communities of practice in the field of physical and mental health, encompassing a diversity of people with general and mental health needs, informal carers and health, social care and education personnel, to establish and connect communities in a mutual or reciprocal fashion to enhance physical and mental health and well-being. It is time to extend beyond a reductive focus on recovery of particular patient groups and conditions. Here, we use the term 'community' advisedly, aware that there are various reductive and even contested definitions of such a term.

As we indicated in Crawford et al. (2013b), this approach is in keeping with a 'new wave of mutuality' and a growing ambition for 'co-operation' (Murray, 2012). Many scholars, for example Tew (2012), have established that social and cultural connectedness can facilitate human recovery. But how much is this key aspect of driving the physical and mental health of populations at the heart of provider business? Clearly, contemporary healthcare provision is most deeply rooted in medical and pharmacological solutions rather than in the contribution of shared community values and participation to such a mutual recovery agenda. Medicine and 'pharma' do not focus explicitly on self-reliance and resilience; nor do they deal with how physical and mental health is 'co-produced' in community settings. Importantly, these dominating pillars to healthcare do not encompass or extend to a vision on how mutual or reciprocal benefits can accrue across and between communities of practitioners, informal carers, patients and the self-caring public. The latter may prove to be the best paradigm for advancing participation, prosperity, sustainability, and health and well-being of societies into a cash-strapped future. At the time of writing, the UK and many other leading countries are faced with austerity measures as well as changing and often challenging demographics. For example, in the UK, the ageing population and rise of dementias is creating a perfect storm threatening sustainability of centralised health and social care services.

With the increasing burden and costs of physical illness, disability and mental distress (see, for example, Centre for Mental Health, 2010; European College of Neuropsychopharmacology, 2009; Wittchen, 2011; World Health Organization (WHO), 2005), a new paradigm for recovery is appearing: what we have referred to as 'mutual recovery'. This has emerged out of the idea of 'recovery' which has developed from civil rights and survivor movements in both the US and UK contexts, most forthrightly in the mental health sector. There is a lot of momentum to this movement which positions people in distress or disability in their social contexts, looks to foreground and build upon their own views of their situation, promotes resilience, and challenges established authorities and communities of expertise. It is about such individuals living fuller lives, having access to employment, education and full citizenship. This model is now gaining ground worldwide, not least in Europe (Department of Health, 2011; WHO, 2005), supported by professional, third sector and activist movements (Boardman and Shepherd, 2009; Shepherd et al., 2008) and congruent with self-help and resilience models (Amering and Schmolke, 2009). Furthermore, it fits an increased focus on social contexts in advancing physical and mental health, for bringing parity between these and for cohering multiple capacities and resources for healthy nations, not least in regard to decent housing, employment and other social capital opportunities.

But this 'recovery' movement is not single-tracked or by any means totalised by any single group of advocates or commentators. Indeed, the notion of 'recovery' has opened up a turbulent field, with various definitions, accommodations and applications of the term. It has contested value as a concept, provoking debate on whose business recovery is. Should this be a grassroots and peer-to-peer movement or something professionally controlled and doled out? Is 'recovery' synonymous or coterminal with 'cure'? It is our view that the notion has utility for various possible social actions based loosely around the definition mooted above but that its most radical potential lies in combination with a philosophy or principle of mutuality. We would contend that it is in this area that the new kinds of institutions, practices, identities, and discourses of 'recovery' will reach full tilt and create across physical and mental health care more future-proof provision of support and cohesion in society.

To summarise for a moment then, co-producing a more resilient life and generating positive social and cultural connections for health and well-being through mutual practices and relationships is something that has implications beyond people with any particular physical or mental health condition. It is driven by a reciprocal or mutual ambit. It seeks to bring health and well-being benefits for all involved in formal and informal healthcare or well-being activity, shifting the focus beyond the individual patient or client recipient to informal carers, health, social care and education personnel. It is here, as will be discussed below, that the compassionate design (Crawford, 2013a) of health and social care can incorporate such notions of mutual recovery in which creative practice could play a major part.

Viewing recovery in this reciprocal way opens up new possibilities for examining how recovery for physical and mental health could occur through a new parity of shared practice within and across these groups or communities, and how creative practice may assist such a mutual process, countering the traditional focus only on individuals more obviously in need, that is patients or clients. It is the latter individualised conceptions of recovery that have emerged within health services and policy thus far. Mutual recovery offers instead a basis around interactional processes, identities and social relationships and is, therefore, a powerfully applicable term because it engages with a deeper social understanding of physical and mental health recovery processes. It is more ambitious in encompassing an array of contributors to physical and mental health.

It is common for people with physical or mental health needs, informal carers and health, social care and allied personnel, for example in education, to be deemed separate or divided individuals, groups or even communities. There is little in the way of comprehensive programmes of work to forge connectivity between such individuals, groups or communities receiving or contributing to physical and mental health and well-being in and through shared creative capital in the visual arts, music, dance, drama, stories/narratives, histories, philosophies and so on.

There is a need to bring together diverse academic and community partners to share insights, approaches, methods and analytic tools in order to mobilise the concept and develop creative practice as mutual recovery to better connect communities for physical and mental health and well-being. Such a move would herald a radical shift in vision in approaches to physical and mental health. It could transform how people with such difficulties, challenges or disabilities, their informal carers, and health, social care and allied personnel in community arts, adult community learning, service user/survivor and carer groups and organisations build together 'egalitarian, appreciative and substantively connected communities – resilient communities of mutual hope, compassion and solidarity' (Crawford et al., 2013b). For too long now, care has been top-heavy with medical/professional rather than community-based solutions. In the case of mental health, for example, the traditional, dominant approaches are deemed flawed (Bentall,

2009) and even the Medical Research Council note 'low research capacity coupled to the perception that the research questions in this field have been relatively intractable' (2010, p. 3). Similarly in physical health and public health, the predominant focus is on evidence based and expressly clinical interventions delivered by experts to individuals or target groups. This suggests that there is fertile ground for innovation. Whilst the recovery movement has spotlighted non-professional solutions and promoted self-help in mental health (Beresford et al., 2010; Davidson et al., 2010; Repper and Perkins, 2003), there is so much more to do. For a start, the emergence of recovery in mental health has led to divergent professionalised and grassroots recovery, privileging of individualised recovery over mutual recovery and a lack of ambition to advance generic models for how delivering physical health and well-being can be a more united, cross-community, reciprocal activity of benefit to all parties.

In order to bring a clearer focus on creative practice as mutual recovery, the chapter will now examine an informal carer-centred approach relevant to creative practice in the health humanities which could advance mutual recovery, and finally, how the development of ideas around 'compassionate design' relate to and extend conceptual application.

Informal Carer-Centred Approaches

There are around 6.5 million people in the UK alone who are informal carers, vastly outnumbering 1.3 million health professionals, and by 2037 there will be around 9 million (Carers UK, 2013). Similarly, in the US, there are 65.7 million informal caregivers – 29 per cent of the US adult population – providing care to someone who is disabled, aged or ill (The National Alliance for Caregiving and AARP, 2009). These individuals are often an underappreciated, barely visible hidden 'workforce', maintaining the health of nations, doing their best with little support (Crawford, 2013a). Healthcare and health professional-delivered solutions are arguably dependent on this currently underappreciated and underrepresented group. Indeed, this large part of any population is playing an important role in health and social care – almost as a backbone underpinning various established health services worldwide.

Case Study 8.1   *'No one cares for the carer'*

A is a woman in her 50s, who has physical health challenges in the form of arthritis in her knees. She has three adult children who live away from home. She is divorced and lives alone. Her mother, *J*, is 84 and was diagnosed with Alzheimer's dementia in 2010. *A* says: 'I knew things were going wrong, but the first psychiatrist we saw refused to ask me my opinion, completed a test and said "she scored 28, she's not got dementia". He very reluctantly agreed to refer her for a brain scan – I was insistent that something was wrong, because when we left the appointment she didn't know where we were or who the doctor we'd just seen was, and when we arrived home 20 minutes later she told me thank you for taking her shopping!' At a return appointment with a different psychiatrist, she was formally diagnosed with advanced Alzheimer's. *A* says: 'I was shocked – I knew she had it, but if I hadn't insisted on the scan we'd have got nowhere!' *J* was then conned several times out of substantial sums of money by a local gang of fraudsters. The police were contacted and referred her as a Vulnerable Adult to Social Services. It took two years – and several more safeguarding incidents – to ensure *J*'s safety in a full-time residential home.

A found professional services to be unhelpful a lot of the time, and – in her words – 'resistant to everything that would involve a cost to them'. She did, however, find great comfort in a local Carer's Cafe, where two important health humanities resources were suggested to her – Michael Ignatieff's novel *Scar Tissue* (1994) and The Reading Agency's Mood Boosting Books scheme for carers (see Chapter 3). This enabled both escapism and knowledge building and a sense that someone understood and captured her experience (in Ignatieff's novel).

When asked what would have helped most, *A* suggested a reading group specially for carers, at the local library. Her experience of caring was that 'no one cared for the carer – I was on my own, even when I went into hospital for surgery. Nothing was offered – we were just told to get a neighbour to check on my Mum and give her medication and dinner. We had to fight all the way and, when I asked for a carer's assessment, no one could agree on who should do it, so I gave up. No one cares for carers.'

Thank you to A. B. for agreeing to her story being shared here – some identifying details have been changed at her request.

In the UK context, whilst a movement from in-patient care to care in the community has been taking place for several decades, what is less clear is how we ensure that those communities, families and social networks are strong, resilient and able to measure up to the complex and challenging caring tasks they are often expected to perform. Yet globally, it is timely, given the frequent political demands to curb state spending on healthcare and the often shared economic threats, that there is a shift in emphasis to robustly underpin the greatest healthcare asset worldwide: informal carers.

Earlier policy in the UK context, such as *Recognised, Valued and Supported* (Department of Health, 2010), *Caring about Carers* (Department of Health, 1999) as well as a good deal of policy and practice by local authorities, together with carers assessments available via the NHS UK and OFSTED's work on young carers and schooling, has moved in the right direction, but it is timely to take stock of the situation, evaluate its operation, and deepen and strengthen the policy steps that have already been taken. Importantly, it is clear that these different organisational approaches need to be brought together under a coherent strategy, getting agencies out of their respective silos. This will require all statutory health and social care providers engaging more fully with informal carers as co-care providers with these organisations, mandating formal and auditable engagements that include more unified or joined-up education/training opportunities both offline and online for carers, and robust peer and social support mechanisms for informal carers. It will need a much stronger focus on how best to work alongside informal carers to advance their health and well-being, develop carer support plans and advance informal carer education to maximise self-, family- and community-solutions. Importantly, we also need to be looking beyond traditional supports for health and well-being and investigate how the arts and humanities can be applied to reduce the burden on informal carers, and afford them access to their own recovery in recovering the lives of loved ones they care for. This is an emergent focus with some charities, for example Artcore in the UK which offers creative breaks for carers, but much more needs to be done.

Regarding health research and development, the involvement of patients, the public, and current- and ex-service users in healthcare research has been a key aim of the UK government for the last five years. Collaborative health research and implementation organisations have been tasked on this. There is scope, however, to broaden the horizon of NHS and health services research and improvement work by also including informal and unpaid health and social care workers. Furthermore these individuals could be prioritised in terms of developing and increasing their access to creative practices from the arts and humanities and innovative engagement with creative communities. To date there has been only minimal focus on how arts and humanities may benefit and sustain informal carers, enhance their health and well-being, and bridge the kind of isolation that can occur, especially when caring for people with long-term and chronic conditions such as dementias in the home environment. Here more innovative inclusions in cultural life through IT-based creative networking and outreach of local arts and humanities initiatives, charitable creative organisations and museums and galleries etc. could be key in reducing the burden of informal-carer citizens and increasing their social connectedness.

Bringing informal carers into a more central position rather than as peripheral to healthcare services and advancing creative resources and involvement with them could prove invaluable. Enhanced cultural connectedness for them could bring much needed respite and relief from the burden of their work, increase their resilience in the face of caring, and break their frequent isolation. This need not be limited to hospital-based activities or integral to community visits to individual households but also available in new creative connections online, especially those which advance a local community development at the same time. It is time to move informal carers centre stage and better connect this major asset for any nation, taking forward the hidden potential for cultural capital to be more impactful in a practical and socially inclusive way.

Both activities referred to in Case Study 8.2 were self-started yet indicate the potential for arts and humanities to make a real difference to the lived experience of informal carers. This is something that should be capitalised upon and developed much further, be it horticultural artistry, online reading groups, itinerant visual and performing art, local history and so on. Yet, to date, much of the application of arts and humanities in healthcare has been in dedicated facilities such as hospitals, often within a therapies frame for patients and clients rather than informal carers and not so well established in diverse community settings.

Case Study 8.2 *A personal case study*

For ten years the former father-in-law of author PC cared for his wife with Alzheimer's disease. For much of this time he did so from the confines of his house and garden. He eventually secured a few hours a week respite care when he could go out more freely and rebuild connections with friends. But this had a minor impact, it seemed, on his own mental health and well-being compared to cultural activities. First, he tended to his garden, presenting it artistically and winning two 'Garden in Bloom' awards in his city. Here, his work within the boundary of his modest property was like an outreach to the community and afforded him with some in-reach of that community at the garden boundary, with positive comments from the passing public and the judges of the competition. In addition, he spent time within the boundary of his house investigating family history.

The focus on how 'mutual recovery as creative practice' applies to informal carers for future solutions in healthcare provision in the UK and globally should be especially attractive to governments attempting to deal with demographic challenges of increasingly older populations or struggling to maintain centralised or anything near comprehensive health and social care over the coming decades. Low-cost reformulations of existing or even currently hidden resources will need to come to the fore together with new mobilisations of arts and humanities institutions and initiatives to impact in the less obvious but vitally important realm of informal care. There are already many carers' groups, and support for carers via established charitable organisations, yet this work could be built on to create a broad-based 'carers' revolution' with a more coherent, visible collective and a much richer engagement with cultural, creative capital.

There needs to be a change in priorities of statutory health and social care organisations to work much more closely and proactively with informal carers for community solutions in the future. In the short term such an approach could deliver an improvement and an effective enhancement to what is currently on offer. In the long term it should be a hugely positive initiative and could even deliver cost savings.

Compassionate Design of Healthcare

We know that the arts can promote 'compassionate spaces' and a 'bonding' social capital (Lewis, 2012a, 2012b; Spandler et al., 2007). Indeed, following some shocking stories of poor care recently in the UK, notoriously in Mid-Staffordshire NHS Trust, there has been great concern about the compassion of healthcare practitioners and the need for compassionate design of services (Brown et al., 2013; Crawford, 2011, 2013b, 2013c; Crawford and Brown, 2011; Crawford and Hallawell, 2011; Crawford et al., 2013a; Kvangarsnes et al., 2014). Such a call for compassionate design of healthcare, ensuring low threat and healthier relationships between people, processes and places, is relevant to 'mutual recovery' and the role of the arts and humanities.

Following the care scandal at Mid-Staffordshire NHS Trust, the UK media generated intense criticism of how key professionals such as nurses have been losing their compassion – acting with coldness, cruelty or disinterest to the suffering of others – sometimes referred to as 'compassion depletion' (Crawford et al., 2013a). This continues to be addressed simplistically as a problem with the individual practitioners, rather than the production-line cold clinics (Crawford and Brown, 2011) and threat cultures (see Gilbert, 2009; Rothschild and Rand, 2006) that health systems in high income societies all too frequently ask practitioners to work in.

Compassion is a highly complex, under-researched concept, often used rhetorically or uncritically, as a kind of 'hurrah word' or, indeed, as a term that is connatural with or that defines nursing. But compassion is not just for nurses or doctors. It is the business of multiple professionals working in healthcare and also of those who manage its services. Importantly it is about the whole system of healthcare delivery, its environments and communities. But we don't hear enough about that. Similarly, the role of creative practices in the arts and humanities within healthcare in generating more compassionate cultures has been underplayed and underutilised. If healthcare environments feel more like dead meat storage units and if practitioners are subject to an unrelenting, high pressure mission to save the public, often under threat of management targets, is it so surprising that compassion dwindles? In response we might consider how arts and humanities could contribute here not just in terms of patient recovery in such sites but also to overall compassionate design of environments for the mutual recovery of all communities, not least practitioners.

Compassion can be defined as being sensitive to the suffering of ourselves and others and having a commitment to do something to relieve it, and we can best capture it in a list of attributes: kind, gentle, warm, loving, affectionate, caring, sensitive, helpful, considerate, sympathetic, comforting, reassuring, calming, open, concerned, empathic, friendly, tolerant, patient, supportive, encouraging, nonjudgemental, understanding, giving, soothing, validating, respectful, attentive. But compassion is not just something that resides in individuals and their moral ambit. It is something that is generated by compassionate environments. The latter is often overlooked and the opportunity to deepen the contribution of creative practices missed in the traditional, highly medicalised paradigms of care. In the spirit of 'mutual recovery' the arts and humanities could assist in advancing the compassionate design of healthcare environments for the benefit of patients, family carers and, importantly, hard-pressed and stressed out practitioners. Although we see seeding of this potential transformation through initiatives such as art, cinema and music in hospitals which may or may not co-involve practitioners, informal carers and patients, much more purposeful shared activity could be developed.

The call for a robust and foregrounded whole system activity of 'compassionate design' of the health services grows out of an increasing body of work that has resulted from recent anxiety about the place of dignity and compassion in healthcare and how to measure or enhance such phenomena. At the King's Fund London, the Point of Care initiative has raised concerns about the damaging impact of the 'target' culture in the NHS UK – the way that modern hospitals resemble factories (Crawford and Brown, 2011). We have yet to see UK or US government policy and organisational change that clearly focuses on how health services (and processes) maximise the likelihood of compassionate relationships and engagement from and among nurses and other clinical and non-clinical staff. If real transformation of hospitals and care homes into compassionate spaces is to occur, it will not be merely through individual practitioners applying the right attributes like some kind of cream. The development of more compassionate health services will need to go deeper than mandating angelic nurses or setting up initiatives for compassion to be poured in as a 'skill' through linear or values-based curricula.

We should all ask that our health services are not turned into production-lines. Our practitioners and our patients should not work or be treated in threat cultures which we know result in compassion fatigue or even moral slide in standards of care. We all deserve more than that. Effectiveness and efficiency in healthcare could, at a stretch, be viewed as compassionate, or even 'practical compassion' (Brown et al., 2013), yet there are untold damages to practitioners and patients in the current bent for factory-style, conveyer belt healthcare. This 'production-line mentality' is so prominent that it is not unusual these days to hear nurses speaking more like factory-supervisors. The rule of the clock or the excuse of being 'far too busy' should not blind us to opportunities to advance compassionate spaces and processes that encourage compassionate relationships. But this is not simply the business of practitioners – that has been the big mistake thus far in debates around compassion. Framing practitioners as less compassionate or lacking compassion is not getting to the point. Compassionate care will be achieved in and by governments and their healthcare organisations designing low-threat, compassion-generating spaces and processes, rather than through spurious 'compassion training' of the workforce.

We need to be promoting compassion from policymakers, harking the evidence on how threat cultures lead to compassion fatigue and guiding real changes in this area by mandating that organisations take seriously 'compassionate design' of services as their key activity and use evidence based management to bring about spaces, processes and resources that are compassionate to practitioners. Only then will we advance the likelihood of practitioners more consistently demonstrating compassion in their approach to patients, and finally, patients in turn showing compassion for hard-pressed practitioners, practitioners to managers and so on.

This reaches into how we adapt the complete architecture of care and its processes – to advance low-threat and supportive spaces for human compassion to thrive. As Martinsen, in her book *Care and Vulnerability*, insists when calling for 'hominess' in clinical settings, the architecture (where we 'dwell'), space and time of healthcare creates particular lived experiences of caring and receiving care which may not be healthy or health-promoting. She writes:

> To dwell is to care, to shelter, so that man may grow and flourish, and gain a foothold in existence... My question is this: does the hospital, with its rooms, corridors and interiors, invite people to dwell in its midst?... Are the rooms productive and useful in such a way that the body is torn from the relations and the rhythms it is in, and permeated and pervaded with rapidity and busyness so that it loses its footing and becomes homeless? (Martinsen, 2006, p. 9)

And later, Martinsen points out that our nurses should not have to care in spaces 'painful to be in, rooms with shameful architecture'. Here, she is not just on about architecture as built environment but the interplay between buildings, space and processes. The revisiting of 'hominess' should be central to new visions, policy and practice in healthcare delivery that we here call 'compassionate design'. There needs to be more emphasis on how the arts and humanities could advance in creative and practical ways the compassionate design of healthcare, transforming and enriching the interactive field of people, processes and spaces. Furthermore, such transformation may come from empowering and encouraging patients, informal carers and health professionals to use the humanising force of arts and humanities to increase the 'hominess' of clinical environments.

During a visit to Sydney, Australia, author PC met a woman who had just been into hospital for further surgery on her brain and heard how she had considered it her responsibility to make the featureless side room she had been allocated as homely and recovery-promoting as possible. 'I wanted to help the surgeon by taking care of myself,' she said, 'by making changes to the space. I brought in my juicer, personalised cushions, pictures and played calming music.' In achieving a compassionate design for her stay in hospital she was surprised to find that practitioners frequently visited her homely space. She felt that they came into her sanctuary for respite from the stressful ward environment. Here, in this example, we get a glimpse of the potential for creative practice as mutual recovery, for a more generous contribution to compassionate design in healthcare. Changes for the good may be best coming from patients and informal carers as much as health professionals or formalised projects.

Summary and Conclusions

In this chapter we propose that much more emphasis should be given not simply to the recovery of patients but to the recovery of informal carers and practitioners, and that creative practice may afford an opportunity for 'mutual recovery' between and across these communities. To date, much of the emphasis of professional care services and professional solutions for health challenges has overlooked the potential contribution of informal carers who make up the very large and hidden 'workforce' behind the health of nations. Access to and involvement in creative practice may be an enabling and supportive force for these individuals. We should look to extend the focus of applied arts and humanities beyond the more traditional therapeutic domain in terms of patient care and recovery and envisage how to advance the health and well-being of informal carers. We propose that creative practice could have a vital role to play in the compassionate design of healthcare to reduce threat, connect communities and benefit practitioners, patients and informal carers. More enlightened managers of health services may do well to consider balancing cold instrumentality, measurement of little but the edges of care and commands for effectiveness and efficiency by exploring such health humanities-led solutions for sustaining and warming up the clinic or ward-based environment, hospital public spaces, primary care centres, and so on. They may take seriously the potential for arts and humanities to build reciprocally 'egalitarian, appreciative and substantively connected communities – resilient communities of mutual hope, compassion and solidarity' (Crawford et al., 2013b).

Concluding Remarks

In this book, we have argued that the majority of healthcare and the generation of health and well-being is non-medical. Despite being a popular activity, visits to the doctor, or doctor consultations in the clinic, are relatively fleeting. Other practitioners and professionals and voluntary sector workers may contribute to care. In hospitals and residential settings clients may spend more time with care assistants, catering and cleaning staff, as well as informal and family carers, than they do with doctors. In other institutions such as schools, prisons and childcare services, roles are changing and a greater degree of responsibility for the mental and physical health of their charges is expected from practitioners. Complementary, alternative healthcare and a strong shift to self-care and community-generated solutions give further notice that medicine and 'medical humanities' is too narrow a bandwidth for considering the contribution that arts and humanities can make to the mental health and well-being of society.

This book has attempted to outline the health humanities as an evolved and more inclusive development beyond medical humanities. The field of medical humanities has grown rapidly in the last decade, but it has not responded to the growing and broadening demand from other professions to become involved, and to accommodate new sectors of the healthcare workforce. As we have described across the different chapters and themes, there are important cohorts of personnel in healthcare, as well as informal carers, who have been largely left out of the medical humanities so far.

Moreover, as different disciplines come to value the contribution made by the arts and humanities and new opportunities emerge in health for the development of new approaches in this field, with research centres and academic programmes for health humanities on the rise, this book can act as a beginning point for new inclusions and new visions. It is an early attempt to outline a fuller range of healthcare and health and well-being activities driven by the arts and humanities.

In distinguishing itself from existing literature in medical humanities which continues to be mostly unidisciplinary, this book has hopefully struck a chord with those wishing for a more inclusive and less medically focused platform for innovative scholarship and healthcare or health and well-being practice. We have proposed to take a broader view of the arts and humanities, rather than being specifically focused on the arts themselves. That is, we have expanded the focus to foreground literary and critical theory, anthropology, linguistics and other social sciences which have a bearing on the issues under discussion. Whereas various literature seeks to explore the arts' role in practice, design and education as it applies to healthcare issues, we have argued for the development of theory, concepts and new ways of understanding. We have shown that there is much work afoot already in the medical humanities, and other healthcare disciplines are developing related approaches, but there is still much work to do in cross-fertilising these activities so as to maximise the benefit to practitioners, informal carers and patients/clients.

Our book has provided the first introductory manifesto for health humanities worldwide and is supplemented by *Health Humanities Reader* (Jones et al., 2014). Together, these publications bring together multiple and expanding fields of enquiry that link health and social care disciplines with the arts and humanities articulated as 'health humanities'. This current book has set out to encourage innovation and novel cross-disciplinary explorations, even in the face of structural and cultural limitations in university and healthcare sectors which tend to promote discrete and over-specialised activities – sometimes maintaining ironically anti-intellectual and damaging hierarchies of knowledge and practice. Although by no means comprehensive or exhaustive, the chapters have foregrounded a range of scholarship and innovative practice available in the field, with special emphasis on the following:

- scholarship based on novel practical initiatives in the health humanities, in training, treatment and support for carers and clients
- a commitment to explore those aspects of healthcare, health and well-being which have hitherto not benefitted from the humanities perspective, such as paramedical and support staff, informal carers and service users
- a thoroughgoing development of critique and critical theory so as to enable readers to question not only current practice but also the foundational assumptions of healthcare and the health humanities themselves
- some radical perspectives on the notion of recovery as a cross-community activity.

Back in 1964, in his book *Crisis in the Humanities*, J. H. Plumb wrote: 'the humanities are at a cross-roads, at a crisis in their existence; they must either change the image that they present, adapt themselves to the needs of a society dominated by science and technology, or retreat into social triviality'. Still today, the humanities remain challenged by the call to social impact and the calls for relevance and utility, not least in relation to the jobs market for graduates. Some, like Stanley Fish (2009), object to moves to shift the humanities into a more pragmatic dimension: 'It is not the business of the humanities to save us, no more than it is their business to bring revenue to a state or a university. What then do they do? They don't do anything, if by "do" is meant bring about effects in the world.' Yet Fish fails to consider the humanities as a mode of survival for humans, generating meaning to life, integral to societal development and sustainability, self and group expression, establishing belonging or trust, and helping to place self and others in contexts or environments. He fails to explore and consider that beyond splendid isolationism there is a big world out there of valuable impacts that can be secured for healthcare, health and well-being by its knowledge and practice.

Health humanities offer a route to impact for the humanities and the subsumed arts. The health humanities movement is a paradigm shift in how arts and humanities can be applied to healthcare, health and well-being. Already, this movement is spreading across the globe and the tradition of medical humanities is changing in response. Major research councils, such as the Arts and Humanities Research Council in the UK, have foregrounded 'health humanities' within their programme of work, other funders of the medical humanities such as the Wellcome Trust have loosened their belts on non-doctor research, and former centres for medical humanities have begun to hybridise into new forms with more inclusive nomenclatures and missions. Whatever the net result of all this going forward, the genetic code of the tradition called 'medical humanities' has been radically altered by the health humanities movement and 'health humanities' looks set to become the superordinate term for the application of arts and humanities to healthcare, health and well-being. This will bring new inclusions, new visions, and ultimately new kinds of society.

References

Abrams, B. (2010) 'Musical therapy?' *Voices: A World Forum for Music Therapy*, www. voices.no/?q=colabrams050410, accessed 13 March 2014.

—— (2011) 'Understanding music as a temporal-aesthetic way of being: Implications for a general theory of music therapy', *Arts in Psychotherapy*, 38:2, 114–119.

—— (2012) 'A relationship-based theory of music therapy: Understanding processes and goals as being-together-musically', in K. E. Bruscia (ed.) *Readings on Music Therapy Theory* (University Park, IL: Barcelona Publishers), pp. 58–76.

—— (2013) 'Music', in K. Kirkland (ed.) *International Dictionary of Music Therapy* (New York: Routledge), pp. 79–80.

Acuna, L. E. (2000) 'Don't cry for us Argentinians: Two decades of teaching medical humanities', *Journal of Medical Ethics: Medical Humanities*, 26, 66–70.

—— (2003) 'Teaching Humanities at the National University of La Plata, Argentina', *Academic Medicine*, 78:10, 1024–1027.

Adamson, E. (1984) *Art as Healing* (London: Coventure).

Adhikari, R. K. (2007) 'Humanities in education of doctors', *Kathmandu University Medical Journal*, 5:20, 443–444.

Adolphs, S., Brown, B., Carter, R., Crawford, P. and Sahota, O. (2004) 'Applying corpus linguistics in a health care context', *Journal of Applied Linguistics*, 1:1, 9–28.

Ahlzen, R. (2007) 'Scientific Contribution: Medical humanities – arts and humanistic science', *Medicine, Health Care and Philosophy*, 10, 385–393.

Ahlzen, R. and Stolt, C. M. (2003) 'The Humanistic Medicine Program at the Karolinska Institute, Stockholm, Sweden', *Academic Medicine*, 78:10, 1039–1042.

Aldridge, D. (1996) *Music Therapy Research and Practice in Medicine: From Out of the Silence* (London: Jessica Kingsley).

—— (2004) *Health, the Individual and Integrated Medicine: Revisiting an Aesthetic of Health Care* (London: Jessica Kingsley).

Aldridge, F. and Dutton, Y. (2009) *Building a Society for All Ages: Benefits for Older People from Learning in Museums, Libraries and Archives* (Leicester: National Institute of Adult Continuing Education/London: Museums, Libraries and Archives Council).

Alford, S., Cheetham, N. and Hauser, D. (2005) *Science and Success in Developing Countries: Holistic Programs that Work to Prevent Teen Pregnancy, HIV, and Sexually Transmitted Infections* (Washington, DC: Advocates for Youth).

Allen, K. N. and Wozniak, K. S. (2014) 'The integration of healing rituals in group treatment for women survivors of domestic violence', *Social Work in Mental Health*, 12, 52–68.

American Association of Medical Colleges (2008) *2008 Annual Report: Creating a Better Tomorrow* (Washington, DC: American Association of Medical Colleges).

American Psychiatric Association (1994) *Diagnostic and Statistical Manual of Mental Disorders* (4th ed. Washington, DC: American Psychiatric Association).

Amering, M. and Schmolke, M. (2009) *Recovery in Mental Health* (Oxford: Wiley-Blackwell).

Amos, T. (1991) *Me and a Gun* [original song].

Andersson, H., Lindholm, C. and Fossum, B. (2011) 'MRSA – global threat and personal disaster: Patients' experiences', *International Nursing Review*, 58:1, 47–53.

Anton, S. (2010) 'Social inclusion through libraries that provide digital health information and support', *Journal of Social Inclusion*, 1:2, 107–110.

Antonovsky, A. (1979) *Health, Stress and Coping* (San Francisco: Jossey-Bass).

—— (1987) *Unraveling the Mystery of Health: How People Manage Stress and Stay Well* (San Francisco: Jossey-Bass).

Argyle, E. and Bolton, G. (2004) 'The use of art within a groupwork setting', *Groupwork*, 14:1, 46–62.

Atkins, S. and Murphy, K. (1993) 'Reflection: A review of the literature', *Journal of Advanced Nursing*, 18:8, 1188–1192.

Austin, D. (2004) *When Words Sing and Music Speaks: A Qualitative Study of In Depth Music Psychotherapy with Adults* (Doctoral dissertation, New York University-UMI Number 3110989).

Baikie, K. A. and Wilhelm, K. (2005) 'Emotional and physical health benefits of expressive writing', *Advances in Psychiatric Treatment*, 11, 338–346.

Baker, C. (2011) '"Nobody's meat": Revisiting rape and sexual trauma through Angela Carter', in S. Onega and J-M. Ganteau (eds) *Ethics and Trauma in Contemporary British Fiction* (Amsterdam and New York: Rodopi), pp. 61–83.

Baker, C., Crawford, P., Brown, B. J., Lipsedge, M. and Carter, R. (2010) *Madness in Post-1945 British and American Fiction* (Basingstoke: Palgrave).

Baker, C., Shaw, C. and Biley, F. (2013) *Our Encounters with Self-Harm* (Ross-on-Wye: PCCS Books).

Baker, P. (2006) *Using Corpora in Discourse Analysis* (London: Continuum).

Bal, M. (1985) *Narratology: Introduction to the Theory of Narrative* (Toronto: University of Toronto Press).

Baldwin, A. (2010) 'Dancing diseases: An applied theatre response to the challenge of conveying emotionally contradictory messages in HIV education', *Applied Theatre researcher/IDEA Journal*, 11, 1–14.

Barclay, M. W. (2007) 'We tell ourselves stories: Psychotherapy and aspects of narrative structure', in S. Krippner, M. Bova and L. Gray (eds) *Healing Stories: The Use of Narrative in Counseling and Psychotherapy* (San Juan, Puerto Rico: Puente), pp. 1–19.

Barthes, R. (1982) 'Introduction to the structural analysis of narratives', in S. Sontag (ed.) *A Barthes Reader* (New York: Hill and Wang), pp. 251–295.

Bates, V., Bleakley, A. and Goodman, S. (eds) (2014) *Medicine, Health and The Arts: Approaches to Medical Humanities* (Oxon: Routledge).

Baudrillard, J. (1983) *Simulations* (trans. by P. Foss, P. Patton and P. Beitchman. New York: Semiotext(e)).

BBC (2002) '"Oldest" prehistoric art unearthed', http://news.bbc.co.uk/1/hi/sci/tech/1753326.stm, accessed 29 March 2014.

BBC (2014) 'Did the trauma of World War One lead to great creativity?', www.bbc.co.uk/guides/zptgq6f, accessed 30 March 2014.

Beard, R. L. (2011) 'Art therapies and dementia care: A systematic review', *Dementia*, DOI: 10.1177/1471301211421090.

Becker, E. and Dusing, S. (2010) 'Participation is possible: A case report of integration into a community performing arts program', *Physiotherapy Theory and Practice*, 26:4, 275–280.

Bell, C. M. (1992) *Ritual Theory, Ritual Practice* (Oxford: Oxford University Press).

—— (1997) *Ritual: Perspectives and Dimensions* (New York: Oxford University Press).

Bentall, R. (2009) *Doctoring the Mind: Why Psychiatric Treatments Fail* (London: Penguin).

Beresford, P., Nettle, M. and Perring, R. (2010) *Towards a Social Model of Madness and Distress? Exploring What Service Users Say* (York: Joseph Rowntree Foundation).

Beveridge, A. (2003) 'Should psychiatrists read fiction?' *British Journal of Psychiatry*, 182, 385–387.

Biley, F. C. and Galvin, K. T. (2007) 'Lifeworld, the arts and mental health nursing', *Journal of Psychiatric and Mental Health Nursing*, 14:8, 800–807.

Bishop, J. P. (2008) 'Rejecting medical humanism: Medical humanities and the metaphysics of medicine', *Journal of Medical Humanities*, 29, 15–25.

Boardman, J. and Shepherd, G. (2009) *Implementing Recovery* (London: Sainsbury Centre for Mental Health).

Boddy, J. (1988) 'Spirits and selves in northern Sudan: The cultural therapeutics of possession and trance', *American Ethnologist*, 15, 427.

Boethius, A. M. S. (1989) *Fundamentals of Music* (ed. by C. V. Palisca, trans. by C. M. Bower. New Haven, CT: Yale University Press).

Bola, J. R. and Mosher, L. R. (2002) 'Clashing ideologies or scientific discourse?' *Schizophrenia Bulletin*, 28:4, 583–588.

Bold, C. (2012) *Using Narrative in Research* (London: Sage).

Bolton, G. (2008) 'Boundaries of humanities: Writing medical humanities', *Arts and Humanities in Higher Education*, 7:2, 131–148.

Bonde, L. O. (2011) 'Health musicing: Music therapy or music and health? A model, empirical examples and personal reflections', *Music and Arts in Action*, 3:2, 120–140.

Bourdieu, P. (1991) *Language and Symbolic Power* (Cambridge: Polity Press).

Bourguignon, E. (1976) *Possession* (San Francisco: Chandler and Sharp).

Boydell, K. M. (2011) 'Making sense of collective events: The co-creation of a research-based dance', *Forum Qualitative Social Research*, 12:1, art. 5, http://nbn-resolving.de/urn:nbn:de:0114-fqs110155, accessed 23 March 2014.

Boydell, K. M., Volpe, T., Cox, S., Katz, A., Dow, R., Brunger, F., et al. (2012) 'Ethical challenges in arts-based health research', *International Journal of*

The Creative Arts in Interdisciplinary Practice, 11, www.ijcaip.com/archives/ IJCAIP-11-paper1. html, accessed 26 March 2014.

Bracken, P. (2007) 'Beyond models, beyond paradigms: The radical interpretation of recovery', in P. Stastny and P. Lehmann (eds) *Alternatives Beyond Psychiatry* (Berlin: Peter Lehman Publishing), pp. 400–402.

Brawer, J. R. (2006) 'The value of a philosophical perspective in teaching the basic medical sciences', *Medical Teacher*, 28:5, 472–474.

Brodzinski, E. (2010) *Theatre in Health and Care* (Basingstoke: Palgrave Macmillan).

Brooke and Kimball (1993) *Fatso* [original song].

Brown, B., Crawford, P. and Hicks, C. (2003) *Evidence Based Research* (Buckingham: Open University Press).

Brown, B., Crawford, P. and Carter, R. (2006) *Evidence-Based Health Communication* (Maidenhead: Open University Press).

Brown, B., Crawford, P., Gilbert, P., Gilbert, J. and Gale, C. (2013) 'Practical compassions: Repertoires of practice and compassion talk in acute mental health', *Sociology of Health and Illness*, 36:3, 383–399.

Brown, B., Tanner, J. and Padley, W. (In press) '"This wound has spoiled everything": Emotional capital and the experience of surgical site infections', *Sociology of Health and Illness*.

Brown, C. and Augusta-Scott, T. (2007) 'Introduction: Postmodernism, reflexivity, and narrative therapy', in C. Brown and T. Augusta-Scott (eds) *Narrative Therapy: Making Meaning, Making Lives* (Thousand Oaks, CA: Sage), pp. ix–xliii.

Brown, P. and De Graaf, S. (2013) 'Considering a future which may not exist: The construction of time and expectations amidst advanced-stage cancer', *Health, Risk and Society*, 15:6–7, 543–560.

Brown, S. and Dissanayake, E. (2009) 'The arts are more than aesthetics: Neuroaesthetics as narrow aesthetics', in M. Skov and O. Vartanian (eds) *Neuroaesthetics* (Amityville: Baywood), pp. 43–57.

Brown, W. and Kandirikirira, N. (2007) *Recovering Mental Health in Scotland: Report on Narrative Investigation of Mental Health Recovery* (Glasgow: Scottish Recovery Network).

Bruner, J. (1990) *Acts of Meaning* (Cambridge, MA: Harvard University Press).

Buber, M. (1971) *I and Thou* (New York: Touchstone).

Burnett, E., Lee, K., Rushmer, R., Ellis, M., Noble, M. and Davey, P. (2010) 'Healthcare-associated infection and the patient experience: A qualitative study using patient interviews', *Journal of Hospital Infection*, 74:1, 42–47.

Butler, J. (1993) *Bodies That Matter: On the Discursive Limits of Sex* (New York: Routledge).

Calman, K. C. (2005) 'The arts and humanities in health and medicine', *Public Health*, 119:11, 958–959.

Camic, P., Tischler, V. and Pearman, C. (2013) 'Viewing and making together: A multi-session art gallery based intervention for people with dementia and their carers', *Aging and Mental Health*, DOI: 10.1080/13607863.2013.818101.

Campbell, J. (1949) *The Hero with a Thousand Faces* (Princeton, NJ: Princeton University Press).

Campbell, M. L. (2012) 'Aesthetics, ambience, and institutional health care environments', *Journal of Palliative Medicine*, 15:10, 1052.

Cardeña, E., van Duijl, M., Weiner, L. and Terhune, D. (2009) 'Possession/trance phenomena', in P. F. Dell and J. A. O'Neil (eds) *Dissociation and the Dissociative Disorders: DSM-V and Beyond* (New York: Routledge), pp. 171–181.

Carers UK (2013) 'Statistics and facts about carers', www.carersuk.org/news room/stats-and-facts, accessed 7 April 2014.

Carey, J. (2006) *What Good are the Arts?* (New York: Faber and Faber).

Carless, D. and Douglas, K. (2010) 'Performance ethnography as an approach to health-related education', *Educational Action Research*, 18:3, 373–388.

Carlson, L. E. and Bultz, B. (2008) 'Mind–body interventions in oncology', *Current Treatment Options in Oncology*, 9, 127–134.

Carr, W. and Kemmis, S. (1986) *Becoming Critical: Knowing through Action Research* (Victoria: Deakin University Press).

Carstairs, G. M. and Kapur, R. L. (1976) *The Great Universe of Kota* (London: Hogarth Press).

Castro, R. (1995) 'The subjective experience of health and illness in Ocuituco: A case study', *Social Science and Medicine*, 41:7, 1005–1021.

Centre for Mental Health (CMH) (2010) *The Economic and Social Costs of Mental Health Problems in 2009/10* (London: CMH).

Chamberlain, D., Heaps, D. and Robert, I. (2008) 'Bibliotherapy and information prescriptions: A summary of the published evidence-base and recommendations from past and ongoing Books on Prescription projects', *Journal of Psychiatric and Mental Health Nursing*, 15:1, 24–36.

Charon, R. (2000) 'Literature and medicine: Origins and destinies', *Academic Medicine*, 75:1, 23–27.

—— (2001) 'Narrative medicine: A model for empathy, reflection, profession, and trust', *Journal of the American Medical Association*, 286:15, 1897–1902.

—— (2006a) 'The self-telling body', *Narrative Inquiry*, 16:1, 191–200.

—— (2006b) *Narrative Medicine: Hearing the Stories of Illness* (Oxford: Oxford University Press).

Chesler, P. (2005) *Women and Madness: Revised and Updated* (New York: Palgrave Macmillan).

Christakis, N. A. (1995) 'The similarity and frequency of proposals to reform US medical education: Constant concerns', *Journal of the American Medical Association*, 274:9, 706–711.

Christie, D., Hood, D. and Griffin, A. (2006) 'Thinking, feeling and moving: Drama and movement therapy as an adjunct to a multidisciplinary rehabilitation approach for chronic pain in two adolescent girls', *Clinical Child Psychology and Psychiatry*, 11:4, 569–577.

Churchill, S. D. (2000) 'Phenomenological psychology', in A. D. Kazdin (ed.) *Encyclopedia of Psychology* (Oxford: Oxford University Press).

Clark, B. (1972) *Whose Life Is It Anyway?* [play].

Clark, H. (2013) *A question that sometimes drives me hazy: Am I, or are the others crazy?* [choreographed dance], www.easyreadernews. com/76034/hermosa-beach-choreographer-tackles-mental-illness/, accessed 23 March 2014.

Clarke, L. (2009) *Fiction's Madness* (Ross-on-Wye: PCCS Books).

Clift, S. and Hancox, G. (2010) 'The significance of choral singing for sustaining psychological wellbeing: Findings from a survey of choristers in England, Australia and Germany', *Music Performance Research*, 3:1, 79–96.

Collett, T. J. and McLachlan, J. C. (2005) 'Does "doing art" inform students' learning of anatomy?', *Medical Education*, 39, 505–533.

Collins, S. (2005) 'Explanations in consultations: The combined effectiveness of doctors' and nurses' communication with patients', *Medical Education*, 39, 785–796.

Conard, N. J., Malina, M. and Münzel, S. C. (2009) 'New flutes document the earliest musical tradition in Southwestern Germany', *Nature*, 460, 737–740.

Cordle, H., Fradgley, K., Carson, J., Holloway, F. and Richards, P. (2011) *Psychosis: Stories of Recovery and Hope* (London: Quay Books).

Crawford, M. J., Killaspy, H., Barnes, T. R. E., Barrett, B., Byford, S., Clayton, K., et al. (2012) 'Group art therapy as an adjunctive treatment for people with schizophrenia: Multicentre pragmatic randomised trial', *British Medical Journal*, 344, e846.

Crawford, P. (2011) 'NHS failures in care for the elderly demand prompt remedies', Letter to the Editor, *The Times*, 14 October, 35.

—— (2013a) 'Compassion is not just for nurses, it's for managers too: Lead article', *Public Servant*, March, 10–11.

—— (2013b) 'Mental health and informal care: Maybe now, finally, we can start polishing our hidden gems', Guest Editorial, *nhsManagers.network*, www.nhs managers. net/guest-editorials/mental-health-and-informal-care-maybe-now-finally-we-can-start-polishing-our-hidden-gems/, accessed 27 March 2014.

—— (2013c) 'The NHS and the true meaning of compassion', *Health and Social Care Reform: GovToday*, Editor's Feature, www.hscreformseries.co.uk/leadership/14747-the-nhs-and-the-true-meaning-of-compassion, accessed 27 March 2014.

Crawford, P. and Baker, C. (2009) 'Literature and madness: A survey of fiction for students and professionals', *Journal of Medical Humanities*, 30, 237–251.

Crawford, P. and Brown, B. (2011) 'Fast healthcare: Brief communication, traps and opportunities', *Patient Education and Counselling*, 82, 3–10.

Crawford, P. and Hallawell, B. (2011) 'Where is the love?' *Learning Disabilities Practice*, 14:6, 9.

Crawford, P., Brown, B. and Nolan, P. (1998) *Communicating Care: The Language of Nursing* (Cheltenham: Stanley Thornes Publishers – A division of the Kluwer Group).

Crawford, R., Brown, B. and Crawford, P. (2004) *Storytelling in Therapy* (Cheltenham: Nelson Thornes).

Crawford, P., Brown, B., Tischler, V. and Baker, C. (2010) 'Health humanities: The future of medical humanities?', *Mental Health Review*, 15:3, 4–10.

Crawford, P., Gilbert, P., Gilbert, J., Gale, C. and Harvey, K. (2013a) 'The language of compassion in acute mental health care', *Qualitative Health Research*, 23:6, 719–727.

Crawford, P., Lewis, L., Brown, B. and Manning, N. (2013b) 'Creative practice as mutual recovery in mental health', *Mental Health Review Journal*, 18:2, 44–64.

Csikszentmihalyi, M. (1997) *Finding Flow: The Psychology of Engagement with Everyday Life* (New York: Basic Books).

Csordas, T. J. (1987) 'Genre, motive and metaphor: Conditions for creativity in ritual language', *Cultural Anthropology*, 2:4, 445–469.

Cunningham, C., Peters, K. and Mannix, J. (2013) 'Physical health inequities in people with severe mental illness: Identifying initiatives for practice change', *Issues in Mental Health Nursing*, 34, 855–862.

Daly, J., Willis, K., Small, R., Green, J., Welch, N., Kealy, M. and Hughes, E. (2007) 'A hierarchy of evidence for assessing qualitative health research', *Journal of Clinical Epidemiology*, 60, 43–49.

Davidson, L., Rakfeldt, J. and Strauss, J. (2010) *The Roots of the Recovery Movement in Psychiatry* (Chichester: Wiley-Blackwell).

Davis, C. (2003) 'Nursing humanities: The time has come', *American Journal of Nursing*, 103, 13.

Davis, J., Tomkins, J. and Roberts, S. (2008) 'A reading revolution on the Wirral', *Public Library Journal*, 23:3, 25–28.

DeFlem, M. (1991) 'Ritual, anti-structure and religion: A discussion of Victor Turner's Processual Symbolic Analysis', *Journal for the Scientific Study of Religion*, 90:1, 1–25.

Deleuze, G. and Guattari, F. (1980) *A Thousand Plateaus* (trans. by Brian Massumi. London and New York: Continuum).

Dellasega, C., Milone-Nuzzo, P., Curci, K., Ballard, J. O. and Kirch, D. G. (2007) 'The humanities interface of nursing and medicine', *Journal of Professional Nursing*, 23:3, 174–179.

DeLuca, C. (2011) 'Interpretive validity theory: Mapping a methodology for validating educational assessments', *Educational Research*, 53:3, 303–320.

Demenaga, M. and Jackson, D. (2010) 'An introduction to art psychotherapy', in V. Tischler (ed.) *Mental Health Psychiatry and the Arts* (London: Radcliffe Publishing), pp. 75–87.

DeNora, T. (2000) *Music in Everyday Life* (Cambridge, UK: Cambridge University Press).

—— (2007) 'Health and music in everyday life: A theory of practice', *Psyke and Logos*, 28:1, 271–287.

Denzin, N. K. (1989) *Interpretive Interactionism* (London: Sage).

—— (1997) *Interpretive Ethnography: Ethnographic Practices in the 21st Century* (Thousand Oaks, CA: Sage).

Department of Health (DH) (1996) *Promoting Clinical Effectiveness: A Framework for Action In and Through the NHS* (London: Department of Health).

—— (1999) *Caring about Carers: A National Strategy for Carers* (London: Department of Health).

—— (2010) *Recognised, Valued and Supported: Next Steps for the Carers Strategy* (London: Department of Health).

—— (2011) *No Health Without Mental Health: A Cross-Government Mental Health Outcomes Strategy for People of All Ages* (Gateway Ref 14679. London: Department of Health).

Devlin, P. (2009) *Restoring the Balance: The Effect of Arts Participation on Wellbeing and Health* (Newcastle-upon-Tyne: Voluntary Arts England).

Dew, K., Chamberlain, K., Hodgetts, D., Norris, P., Radley, A. and Gabe, J. (2014) 'Home as a hybrid centre of medication practice', *Sociology of Health and Illness*, 36:1, 28–43.

Di Benedetto, M., Lindner, H., Aucote, H., Churcher, J., McKenzie, S., Croning, N. and Jenkins, E. (2014) 'Co-morbid depression and chronic illness related to coping and physical and mental health status', *Psychology, Health and Medicine*, 19:3, 253–262.

Diekman, A. B., McDonald, M. and Gardner, W. L. (2000) 'Love means never having to be careful: The relationship between reading romance novels and safe sex behaviour', *Psychology of Women Quarterly*, 24:2, 179–188.

Dissanayake, E. (1992) *Homo Aestheticus: Where Art Comes From and Why* (New York: Free Press).

—— (2000) *Art and Intimacy: How the Arts Began* (Seattle: University of Washington Press).

—— (2001) 'An ethological view of music and its relevance for music therapy', *Nordic Journal of Music Therapy*, 10:2, 159–175.

—— (2009) 'The artification hypothesis and its relevance to cognitive science, evolutionary aesthetics, and neuroaesthetics', *Cognitive Semiotics*, 5, 148–173.

Donohoe, M. and Danielson, S. (2004) 'A community-based approach to the medical humanities', *Medical Education*, 38:2, 204–217.

Driver, T. (1998) *Liberating Rites: Understanding the Transformative Power of Ritual* (Boulder, CO: Westview Press).

Duursma, E., Augustyn, M. and Zuckerman, B. (2008) 'Reading aloud to children: The evidence', *Archives of Disease in Childhood*, 93:7, 554–557.

Dysart-Gale, D. (2008) 'Lost in translation: Bibliotherapy and evidence-based medicine', *Journal of Medical Humanities*, 29:1, 33–43.

Dzokkoto, V. A. and Adams, G. (2005) 'Understanding genital-shrinking epidemics in West Africa: koro, juju or mass psychogenic illness?' *Culture, Medicine and Psychiatry*, 29:3, 53–78.

Eaglestone, R. (2009) *Doing English* (London: Routledge).

Eberle, T. S. (2010) 'The phenomenological life-world analysis and the methodology of the social sciences', *Human Studies*, 33, 123–139.

Edson, M. (1995) *Wit* [play].

Edwards, D. (2004) *Art Therapy* (Thousand Oaks, CA: Sage).

Edwards, D., Burnard, P., Coyle, D., Fothergill, A. and Hannigan, B. (2000) 'Stress and burnout in community mental health nursing: A review of the literature', *Journal of Psychiatric and Mental Health Nursing*, 7:1, 7–14.

Eekelaar, C., Camic, P. and Springham, N. (2012) 'Art galleries, episodic memory and verbal fluency in dementia: An exploratory study', *Psychology of Aesthetics, Creativity, and the Arts*, 6, 262–272.

Efland, A (1990) *A History of Art Education: Intellectual and Social Currents in Teaching the Visual Arts* (New York: Teachers College Press).

Eliade, M. (1964) *Shamanism: Archaic Techniques of Ecstasy* (Princeton, NJ: Princeton University Press).

Elliott, D. J. (1995) *Music Matters: A New Philosophy of Music Education* (New York: Oxford University Press).

Enarson, C. and Burg, F. D. (1992) 'An overview of reform initiatives in medical education 1906 through 1992', *Journal of the American Medical Association*, 268:9, 1141–1143.

Eugenides, J. (1993) *The Virgin Suicides* (London: Abacus, 2001).

European College of Neuropsychopharmacology (ECNP) (2009) 22nd Congress, 12 September 2009, Istanbul.

Evans, M. (2003) 'Roles for literature in medical education', *Advances in Psychiatric Treatment*, 9, 380–386.

Fatovic-Ferencic, S. (2003) 'The history of medicine teaching program in Croatia', *Academic Medicine*, 78:10, 1028–1030.

Favazza, A. (1996) *Bodies Under Siege: Self-Mutilation and Body Modification in Culture* (Baltimore: The John Hopkins University Press).

Feder, L. (1980) *Madness in Literature* (Princeton, NJ: Princeton University Press).

Felman, S. (1985) *Writing and Madness (Literature/Philosophy/Psychoanalysis)* (trans. by M. Noel Evans. California: Stanford University Press, 2003).

Fergusson, F. (1968) *The Idea of a Theatre: A Study of Ten Plays, the Art of Drama in Changing Perspective* (Princeton, NJ: Princeton University Press).

Ferrell, B., Virani, R., Jacobs, H. H., Malloy, P. and Kelly, K. (2010) 'Arts and humanities in palliative nursing education', *Journal of Pain and Symptom Management*, 39:5, 941–945.

Finlay, L. (2007) 'Qualitative research towards public health', in S. Earle (ed.) *Theory and Research in Promoting Public Health* (London: Sage).

Fish, S. (2009) 'Will the humanities save us?', http://opinionator.blogs.nytimes.com/2008/01/06/will-the-humanities-save-us/ accessed 1 December 2010.

Floyd, M. (2003) 'Bibliotherapy as an adjunct to psychotherapy for depression in older adults', *Journal of Clinical Psychology*, 59:2, 187–195.

Fonseca, J. (2004) *Contemporary Psychodrama: New Approaches to Theory and Technique* (New York: Psychology Press).

Forsyth, R. and Jarvis, S. (2002) 'Participation in childhood', *Child: Care Health and Development*, 28:4, 277–279.

Fox, N. (2003) 'Practice based evidence: Towards collaborative and transgressive research', *Sociology*, 37, 81–102.

Frame, J. (1961) *Faces in the Water* (London: The Women's Press, 1996).

Frank, A. (1995) *The Wounded Storyteller: Body, Illness, and Ethics* (Chicago, IL: University of Chicago Press).

Frank, A. W. (2003) 'Survivorship as craft and conviction: Reflections on research in progress', *Qualitative Health Research*, 13, 247–255.

Fraser, K. D. and al Sayah, F. (2011) 'Arts-based methods in health research: A systematic review of the literature', *Arts and Health: An International Journal for Research, Policy and Practice*, 3, 110–145.

Freedman, K. (2003) *Teaching Visual Culture: Curriculum, Aesthetics, and the Social Life of Art* (New York: Teachers College Press).

Frei, J., Alvarez, S. E. and Alexander, M. B. (2010) 'Ways of seeing: Using the visual arts in nursing education', *Journal of Nursing Education*, 49:12, 672–676.

Frich, J. C. and Fugelli, P. (2003) 'Medicine and the arts in the undergraduate medical curriculum at the University of Oslo Faculty of Medicine, Oslo, Norway', *Academic Medicine*, 78:10, 1036–1038.

Frid, I., Ohlén, J. and Bergbom, I. (2000) 'On the use of narratives in nursing research', *Journal of Advanced Nursing*, 32:3, 695–703.

Frieswijk, N., Steverink, N., Buunk, B. P. and Slaets, J. P. J. (2006) 'The effectiveness of bibliotherapy in increasing the self-management ability of slightly to moderately frail older people', *Patient Education and Counselling*, 61:2, 219–227.

Frude, N. J. (2004) 'Bibliotherapy as a means of delivering psychological therapy', *Clinical Psychology*, 39, 8–10.

Furman, R. (2006) 'Poetic forms and structures in qualitative health research', *Qualitative Health Research*, 16:4, 560–566.

Garden, R. (2009) 'Expanding clinical empathy: An activist perspective', *Journal of General Internal Medicine*, 24:1, 122–125.

Gardner, G. and Cook, R. (2004) 'Telling accounts of wound infections: Avoidance, anomaly and ambiguity', *Health*, 8, 183–197.

Gelsthorpe, L. (1992) 'Response to Martyn Hammersley's paper "On Feminist Methodology"', *Sociology*, 26, 213–218.

Gendlin, E. T. (1997) *Experiencing and the Creation of Meaning* (Evanston, IL: Northwestern University Press).

General Medical Council (1993) *Tomorrow's Doctors: Recommendations on Undergraduate Medical Education* (London: General Medical Council).

Giddens, A. (1991) *Modernity and Self Identity: Self and Society in the Late Modern Age* (Cambridge: Polity).

Gilbert, P. (2009) *The Compassionate Mind* (London: Constable Robinson).

Gilbert, S. M. and Gubar, S. (2000) *The Madwoman in the Attic: The Woman Writer and the Nineteenth Century Literary Imagination* (2nd ed. New Haven and London: Yale University Press).

Gillis, C. M. (2008) 'Medicine and humanities: Voicing connections', *Journal of Medical Humanities*, 29:1, 5–14.

Given, L. M. (ed.) (2008) *The Sage Encyclopedia of Qualitative Research Methods* (Thousand Oaks, CA: Sage).

Goodill, S. (2005) *An Introduction to Medical Dance/Movement Therapy: Health Care in Motion* (London: Jessica Kingsley).

Gordon, J. J. (2005) 'Medical humanities: To cure sometimes, to relieve often, to comfort always', *Medical Journal of Australia*, 182:1, 5–8.

—— (2008) 'Medical humanities: State of the heart', *Medical Education*, 42:4, 333–337.

Goulding, A. (2013) 'How can contemporary art contribute toward the development of social and cultural capital for people aged 64 and older?', *The Gerontologist*, 53:6, 1009–1019.

Grant, A., Biley, F. and Walker, H. (2011) *Our Encounters with Madness* (Ross-on-Wye: PCCS Books).

Grant, A., Haire, J., Biley, F. and Stone, B. (2013) *Our Encounters with Suicide* (Ross-on-Wye: PCCS Books).

Gray, R. E., Fergus, K. D. and Fitch, M. I. (2005) 'Two Black men with prostate cancer: A narrative approach', *British Journal of Health Psychology*, 10, 71–84.

Green, M. C. and Brock, T. C. (1996) 'Mechanisms of narrative persuasion', *International Journal of Psychology*, 31, 13–14.

Greenhalgh, T. and Hurwitz, B. (eds) (1998) *Narrative Based Medicine: Dialogue and Discourse in Clinical Practice* (London: BMJ Books).

—— (1999) 'Narrative based medicine: Why study narrative?' *British Medical Journal*, 318:7175, 48–50.

Guarnaccia, P. J. and Rogler, L. H. (1999) 'Research on culture-bound syndromes: New directions', *American Journal of Psychiatry*, 156, 1322–1327.

Hamkins, S. (2014) *The Art of Narrative Psychiatry* (Oxford: Oxford University Press).

Hammersley, M. (1992) *What's Wrong with Ethnography? Methodological Explorations* (London: Routledge).

Hanna, J. L. (1987) *To Dance is Human: A Theory of Nonverbal Communication* (Chicago, IL: University of Chicago Press).

Hannigan, B. (2001) 'A discussion of the strengths and weaknesses of "reflection" in nursing practice and education', *Journal of Clinical Nursing*, 10, 278–283.

Hanquinet, L. (2013) 'Visitors to modern and contemporary art museums: Towards a new sociology of "cultural profiles"', *The Sociological Review*, 61:4, 790–813.

Harper, E. B. (1963) 'Spirit possession and social structure', in B. Ratman (ed.) *Anthropology on the March* (London: Oxford University Press), pp. 56–62.

Harvey, G. and Wallis, R. J. (2007) *Historical Dictionary of Shamanism (Historical Dictionaries of Religions, Philosophies, and Movements Series*, No. 77. Latham, MD: The Scarecrow Press).

Harvey, K. and Brown, B., (2012) 'Health communication and psychological distress: Exploring the language of self-harm', *Canadian Modern Language Review*, 68:3, 316–340.

Harvey, K., Brown, B., Crawford, P., Macfarlane, A. and McPherson, A. (2007) '"Am I normal?": Teenagers, sexual health and the internet', *Social Science and Medicine*, 65, 771–781.

Hawkins, A. H. (1993) *Reconstructing Illness: Studies in Pathography* (Indiana: Perdue University Press).

—— (1999) 'Pathography: Patient narratives of illness', *The Western Journal of Medicine*, 171, 127–129.

Heidegger, M. (1962) *Being and Time* (rev. ed. New York: Harper and Row).

Hemmings, C. P. (2005) 'Rethinking medical anthropology: How anthropology is failing medicine', *Anthropology and Medicine*, 12:2, 91–103.

Hervey, L. W. (2000) *Artistic Inquiry in Dance/Movement Therapy: Creative Alternatives for Research* (Springfield, IL: Charles C. Thomas).

Hicks, D. (2006) *An Audit of Bibliotherapy/Books on Prescription Activity in England* (London: Arts Council England/Museums, Libraries and Archives Council).

Hicks, D., Creaser, C., Greenwood, H., Spezi, V., White, S. and Frude, N. (2010) 'Public library activity in the areas of health and wellbeing'

(London: Museums, Libraries and Archives Council), www.research.mla.gov.uk/evidence/view-publication.php?dm=nrmandpubid=1068, accessed 1 December 2010.

Hinder, S. and Greenhalgh, T. (2012) '"This does my head in": Ethnographic study of self-management by people with diabetes', *BMC Health Services Research*, 12, 83. www.biomedcentral.com/1472-6963/12/83, accessed 31 March 2014.

Hinton, D., Peou, S., Joshi, S., Nickerson, A. and Simon, N. M. (2013) 'Normal grief and complicated bereavement among traumatized Cambodian refugees: Cultural context and the central role of dreams of the dead', *Culture, Medicine and Psychiatry*, 37:3, 427–464.

Ho, A. H. Y., Leung, P. P. Y., Tse, D. M. W., Pang, S. M. C., Chochinov, H. M., Neimeyer, R. A. and Chan, C. L. W. (2013) 'Dignity amidst liminality: Healing within suffering among Chinese terminal cancer patients', *Death Studies*, 37, 953–970.

Hodge, S., Robinson, J. and Davis, P. (2007) 'Reading between the lines: The experiences of taking part in a community reading project', *Medical Humanities*, 33, 100–104.

Hogan, S. (2002) *Healing Arts* (London: Jessica Kingsley).

Holloway, I. and Freshwater, D. (2007a) 'Vulnerable story telling: Narrative research in nursing', *Journal of Research in Nursing*, 12, 703–711.

—— (2007b) *Narrative Research in Nursing* (Oxford: Blackwell).

Holmwood, J. (1995) 'Feminism and epistemology: What kind of successor science?' *Sociology*, 29, 411–428.

Horne, O. and Csipke, E. (2009) 'From feeling too little and too much, to feeling more and less? A nonparadoxical theory of the functions of self-harm', *Qualitative Health Research*, 19, 655–667.

Hornstein, G. A. (2012) *Agnes's Jacket: A Psychologist's Search for the Meanings of Madness* (Ross-on-Wye: PCCS Books).

Huskinson, L. (2010) 'Analytical psychology and spirit possession: Towards a nonpathological diagnosis of spirit possession', in B. A. Schmidt and L. Huskinson (eds) *Spirit Possession and Trance* (New York: Continuum International), pp. 71–96.

Hwang, K., Fan, H. and Hwang, S. W. (2013) 'Writing about an experience of illness in medical students', *Advances in Medical Education and Practice*, 4, 151–155.

Ignatieff, M. (1994) *Scar Tissue* (London: Vintage).

Institute of Mental Health (2014) 'Art at the Institute', www.institutemh.org.uk/x-about-us-x/art-at-the-institute, accessed 29 March 2014.

Jameson, F. (1991) *Postmodernism or, The Cultural Logic of Late Capitalism* (London: Verso).

Jamison, C. and Scogin, F. (1995) 'The outcome of cognitive bibliotherapy with depressed adults', *Journal of Consulting and Clinical Psychology*, 63:4, 644–650.

Jones, J. M. (2000) '"The falling sickness" in literature', *Southern Medical Journal*, 93:12, 1169–1172.

Jones, T., Wear, D., Friedman, L. D. and Vonnegut, M. (eds) (2014) *Health Humanities Reader* (New Jersey: Rutgers University Press).

Joshi, M. V. (2008) 'Medical Humanities Collection Development: Policy Guidelines for Indian Hospital Libraries, World Library and Information Congress: 74th IFLA General Congress and Council', www.ifla.org/IV/ifla74/papers/124-Joshi-en.pdf, accessed 27 March 2014.

Jutel, A. (2008) 'Beyond evidence-based nursing: Tools for practice', *Journal of Nursing Management*, 16:4, 417–421.

Kaiser, K. (2008) 'The meaning of the survivor identity for women with breast cancer', *Social Science and Medicine*, 67, 79–87.

Karkabi, K. and Castel, O. C. (2013) 'Arts in medical education', *Journal of Applied Arts & Health*, 4:3, 355–362.

Kassing, G. (2007) *History of Dance: An Interactive Arts Approach* (rev. ed. Champaign, IL: Human Kinetics).

Kaysen, S. (1993) *Girl, Interrupted* (New York: Random House).

Keitel, E. (1989) *Reading Psychosis: Readers, Texts and Psychoanalysis* (Oxford: Basil Blackwell).

Kempler, N. (2003) 'Finding our voice through poetry and psychotherapy', *Journal of Poetry Therapy*, 16:4, 217–220.

Kersten, P., Ellis-Hill, C., McPherson, K. M. and Harrington, R. (2010) 'Beyond the RCT: Understanding the relationship between interventions, individuals and outcome – the example of neurological rehabilitation', *Disability and Rehabilitation*, 32:12, 1028–1034.

Kettlewell, C. (1999) *Skin Game* (New York: St Martin's Press).

Kiessling, C., Muller, T., Becker-Witt, C., Begenau, J., Prinz, V. and Schleiermacher, S. (2003) 'A Medical Humanities Special Study Module on Principles of Medical Theory and Practice at the Charité, Humboldt University, Berlin, Germany', *Academic Medicine*, 78:10, 1031–1035.

Kinghorn, W. A. (2011) 'Whose disorder?: A constructive MacIntyrean critique of psychiatric nosology', *Journal of Medicine and Philosophy*, 36, 187–205.

Kleinman, A. (1988a) *Rethinking Psychiatry: From Cultural Category to Personal Experience* (New York: Free Press).

—— (1988b) *The Illness Narratives: Suffering, Healing and the Human Condition* (New York: Basic Books).

—— (1998) *The Illness Narratives: Suffering, Healing and the Human Condition* (New York: Basic Books).

Kleinman, A., Eisenberg, L. and Good, B. (1978) 'Culture, illness, and care: Clinical lessons from anthropologic and cross-cultural research', *Annals of Internal Medicine*, 88, 251–258.

Koss-Chioino, J. D. (2006) 'Spiritual transformation, relation and radical empathy: Core components of the ritual healing process', *Transcultural Psychiatry*, 43:4, 652–670.

Krippner, S. (1997) 'Dissociation in many times and places', in S. Krippner and S. Powers (eds) *Broken Images, Broken Selves: Dissociative Narratives in Clinical Practice* (Washington, DC: Brunner-Mazel), pp. 3–40.

Kvale, S. (1996) *InterViews: An Introduction to Qualitative Research Interviewing* (Thousand Oaks, CA: Sage).

Kvangarsnes, M., Torheim, H., Hole, T. and Crawford, P. (2014) 'Nurses' perspectives on compassionate care for patients with exacerbated chronic

obstructive pulmonary disease', *Journal of Allergy and Therapy*, 4:158, DOI: 10.4172/2155-6121.1000158.

Kwan, S. S. (2007) 'Clinical efficacy of ritual healing and pastoral ministry', *Pastoral Psychology*, 55:6, 741–749.

Labov, W. and Waletzky, J. (1967) 'Narrative analysis: Oral versions of personal experience', in J. Helm (ed.) *Essays on the Verbal and Visual Arts* (Seattle: University of Washington Press), pp. 12–44.

La Cour, P. and Hvidt, N. C. (2010) 'Research on meaning-making and health in secular society: Secular, spiritual and religious existential orientations', *Social Science and Medicine*, 71:7, 1292–1299.

Lambek, M. (1980) 'Spirits and spouses: Possession as a system of communication among the Malagasy speakers of Mayotte', *American Ethnologist*, 7, 318–331.

Lambert, H. and McKevitt, C. (2002) 'Anthropology in health research: From qualitative methods to multidisciplinarity', *British Medical Journal*, 325, 210–213.

Langley, D. (2006) *An Introduction to Dramatherapy* (London: Sage).

Lather, P. (1993) 'Fertile obsession: Validity after Post-structuralism', *Sociological Quarterly*, 34, 673–693.

Ledwith, M. (2007) 'On being critical: Uniting theory and practice through emancipatory action research', *Educational Action Research*, 15:4, 597–611.

Lefevre, M. (2004) 'Playing with sound: The therapeutic use of music in direct work with children', *Child and Family Social Work*, 9:4, 333–345.

Lewis, L. (2012a) *'You become a person again': Situated Resilience through Mental Health*. ACL, Research Report, March.

—— (2012b) 'The capabilities approach, adult and community learning and mental health', *Community Development Journal special issue on mental health and community development*, 47:4, 522–537.

Lewis-Fernandez, R. (1994) 'Culture and dissociation: A comparison of ataque de nervios among Puerto Ricans and possession syndrome in India', in D. Spiegel (ed.) *Dissociation: Culture, Mind and Body* (Washington, DC: American Psychiatric Press), pp. 123–167.

Liebmann, M. (2004) *Art Therapy for Groups: A Handbook of Themes and Exercises* (London: Psychology Press).

Lim, K. H., Morris, J. and Craik, C. (2007) 'Inpatients' perspectives of occupational therapy in acute mental health', *Australian Occupational Therapy Journal*, 54:1, 22–32.

Lodge, D. (2002) *Consciousness and the Novel* (London: Secker and Warburg).

Lorde, A. (1980). *The Cancer Journals* (San Francisco: Aunt Lute Books).

Louis-Courvoisier, M. (2003) 'Medical Humanities: A new undergraduate teaching program at the University of Geneva School of Medicine, Switzerland', *Academic Medicine*, 78:10, 1043–1047.

Lucock, M., Leach, C., Iveson, S., Lynch, K., Horsefield, C. and Hall, P. (2003) 'A systematic approach to practice-based evidence in a psychological therapies service', *Clinical Psychology and Psychotherapy*, 10:6, 389–399.

MacDougall, J. and Yoder, P. S. (1998) *Contaminating Theatre: Intersections of Theatre, Therapy, and Public Health* (Evanston, IL: Northwestern University Press).

MacNaughton, J. (2007) 'Art in hospital spaces', *International Journal of Cultural Policy*, 13:1, 85–101.

Madill, A., Jordan, A. and Shirley, C. (2000) 'Objectivity and reliability in qualitative analysis: Realist, contextualist and radical constructionist epistemologies', *British Journal of Psychology*, 91:1, 1–20.

Malchiodi, C. A. (2006) *Expressive Therapies* (New York: Guilford Press).

Malinowski, B. (1997) 'Ritual', in T. Barfield (ed.) *The Dictionary of Anthropology* (Oxford, England: Blackwell Publishing), pp. 410–411.

Malloch, S. and Trevarthan, C. (2010) *Communicative Musicality: Exploring the Basis of Human Companionship* (Oxford: Oxford University Press).

Margison, F., McGrath, G., Barkham, M., Mellor, J., Audin, K., Connoll, J. and Evans, C. (2000) 'Measurement and psychotherapy: Evidence-based practice and practice-based evidence', *The British Journal of Psychiatry*, 177, 123–130.

Marroquín, S. (2012) *The materiality of impermanence* [choreographed dance], www. austin360.com/news/entertainment/arts-theater/dancer-uses-illness-as-creative-muse-2/nRk7r/, accessed 23 March 2014.

Marshall, R. J. (2005) 'Knowledge is a call to action', *Medical Education*, 39, 978–979.

Martinsen, K. (2006) *Care and Vulnerability* (Oslo: Akribe).

Maslow, A. (1954) *Motivation and Personality* (New York: Harper).

Matarasso, F. (2012) *Winter Fires: Art and Agency in Old Age* (London: The Baring Foundation).

Mattelaer, J. J. and Jilek, W. (2007) 'Koro? The psychological disappearance of the penis', *The Journal of Sexual Medicine*, 4:5, 1509–1515.

Mazza, N. (2003) *Poetry Therapy: Theory and Practice* (London: Routledge).

McCarthy, M. and Handford, M. (2004) '"Invisible to us": A preliminary corpus-based study of spoken business English', in U. Connor and T. Upton (eds) *Discourse in the Professions: Perspectives from Corpus Linguistics* (Amsterdam: John Benjamins).

McDonald, L. (ed.) (2004) *Florence Nightingale on Public Health Care: The Collected Works of Florence Nightingale, Vol. 6* (Waterloo, Ontario: Wilfred Laurier University Press).

McElroy, A. and Townsend, P. K. (1989) *Medical Anthropology in Ecological Perspective* (2nd ed. Boulder: Westview Press).

McGrath, P. (1990) *Spider* (London: Penguin, 2002).

McKenna, P. and Haste, E. (1999) 'Clinical effectiveness of dramatherapy in the recovery from neuro-trauma', *Disability and Rehabilitation*, 21:4, 162–174.

McKie, A. and Gass, J. P. (2001) 'Understanding mental health through reading selected literature sources: An evaluation', *Nurse Education Today*, 21, 201–208.

McKie, A., Adams, V., Gass, J. P. and Macduff, C. (2008) 'Windows and mirrors: Reflections of a module team teaching the arts in nurse education', *Nurse Education in Practice*, 8, 156–164.

McLean, C. L. (2014) *Creative Arts in Humane Medicine* (Edmonton, Alberta: Brush Education Inc).

McLeod, J. (2000) *Qualitative Research in Counselling and Psychotherapy* (London: Sage).

McNiff, S. (1998) *Art-Based Research* (London: Jessica Kingsley).

—— (2008) 'Art-based research', in J. G. Knowles and A. L. Cole (eds) *Handbook of the Arts in Qualitative Research: Perspectives, Methodologies, Examples, and Issues* (Thousand Oaks, CA: Sage), pp. 29–40.

Medical Research Council (MRC) (2008) *Developing and Evaluating Complex Interventions: New Guidance* (London: Medical Research Council).

—— (2010) *Review of Mental Health Research* (London: Medical Research Council).

Melley, T. (2000) *Empire of Conspiracy: The Culture of Paranoia in Postwar America* (Ithaca and London: Cornell University Press).

Merleau-Ponty, M. (1962) *Phenomenology of Perception* (London: Routledge and Kegan Paul).

Mienczakowski, J. (1999) 'Ethnography in the hands of participants: Tools of dramatic discovery', *Studies in Educational Ethnography*, 28, 145–161.

Milligan, M. (2012) *Mercy Killers* [play]. http://mercykillerstheplay.com/home/, accessed 24 March 2014.

Mitchell, G., Jonas-Simpson, C. and Ivonoffski, V. (2006) 'Research based theatre: The making of *I'm still here*', *Nursing Science Quarterly*, 19, 198–206.

Moss, H. and O'Neill, D. (2014) 'The aesthetic and cultural interests of patients attending an acute hospital: A phenomenological study', *Journal of Advanced Nursing*, 70:1, 121–129.

Moss, H., Donnellan, C. and O'Neill, D. (2012) 'A review of qualitative methodologies used to explore patient perceptions of arts in healthcare', *Medical Humanities*, 38:2, 106–109.

Moss, P. A. (1996) 'Enlarging the dialogue in educational measurement: Voices from interpretive research traditions', *Educational Researcher*, 25, 20–28.

Murphy, N. A. and Carbone, P. S. (2008) 'Promoting the participation of children with disabilities in sports, recreation, and physical activities', *Pediatrics*, 121, 1057–1061.

Murray, R. (2012) *The New Wave of Mutuality: Social Innovation and Public Service Reform* (London: Policy Network).

Murray, R., McKay, E., Thompson, S. and Donald, M. (2000) 'Practising reflection: A medical humanities approach to occupational therapist education', *Medical Teacher*, 22:3, 276–281.

Nancy, J-L. (2000) *Being Singular Plural* (Palo Alto, CA: Stanford University Press).

National Institute for Health and Clinical Excellence (NICE) (2004) *Clinical Guidelines for the Management of Anxiety: Management of anxiety (panic disorder, with or without agoraphobia, and generalised anxiety disorder) in adults in primary, secondary and community care* (London: National Institute for Health and Clinical Excellence).

Newman, A., Goulding, A. and Whitehead, C. (2012) 'The consumption of contemporary visual art: Identity formation in late adulthood', *Cultural Trends*, 21:1, 29–45.

Noblit, G. W. and Hare, R. D. (1988) *MetaEthnography: Synthesising Qualitative Studies* (Newbury Park, CA: Sage).

Noy, P. and Noy-Sharav, D. (2013) 'Art and emotions', *International Journal of Applied Psychoanalytic Studies*, 10:2, 100–107.

Oakley, A. (1991) 'Interviewing women: A contradiction in terms?' in H. Roberts (ed.) *Doing Feminist Research* (2nd ed. London: Routledge), pp. 30–61.

—— (1998) 'Gender, methodology and people's ways of knowing: Some problems with feminism and the paradigm debate in social science', *Sociology*, 32, 707–731.

O'Donnell, P. (2000) *Latent Destinies: Cultural Paranoia and Contemporary U. S. Narrative* (Durham and London: Duke University Press).

Ola, B. A., Morakinyo, O. and Adewuya, A. O. (2009) 'Brain fag syndrome: A myth or a reality', *African Journal of Psychiatry*, 12:2, 135–143.

Olthuis, G. and Dekkers, W. (2003) 'Medical education, palliative care and moral attitude: Some objectives and future perspectives', *Medical Education*, 37, 928–933.

Ong, A. (1987) *Spirits of Resistance and Capitalist Discipline: Factory Women in Malaysia* (Albany: State University of New York Press).

Online Etymology Dictionary (n.d.) 'Health', http://dictionary.reference.com/browse/health, accessed 13 March 2014.

Onstage Dance Company (2012) 'Dancing about the experience of cancer', http://onstagedanceco.com/1/post/2012/12/dancing-about cancer. html, accessed 16 March 2014.

Osler, W. (1920) *The Old Humanities and the New Science* (Boston: Houghton Mifflin).

Overcash, J. A. (2004) 'Narrative research: A viable methodology for clinical nursing', *Nursing Forum*, 39:1, 15–22.

Oyebode, F. (ed.) (2009) *Mindreadings: Literature and Psychiatry* (London: Royal College of Psychiatry).

Paintings in Hospitals (2014) www.paintingsinhospitals.org.uk/evidence/background, accessed 13 March 2014.

Paley, J. and Eva, G. (2005) 'Narrative vigilance: The analysis of stories in health care', *Nursing Philosophy*, 6, 83–97.

Payne, H. (2004) 'Becoming a client, becoming a practitioner: Student narratives of a dance movement therapy group', *British Journal of Guidance and Counselling*, 32:4, 511–532.

Perry, C., Thurston, M. and Osborn, T. (2008) 'Time for me: The arts as therapy in postnatal depression', *Complementary Therapies in Clinical Practice*, 14, 38–45.

Petersen, A., Bleakley, A., Brömer, R. and Marshall, R. (2008) 'The medical humanities today: Humane health care or tool of governance?' *Journal of Medical Humanities*, 29:1, 1–4.

Pfister, M. (1977) *The Theory and Analysis of Drama* (trans. by J. Halliday. Cambridge, UK: Cambridge University Press European Studies in English Literature Series).

Phillips, P. S. (2000) 'Running a life drawing class for pre-clinical medical students', *Medical Education*, 34, 1020–1025.

Pinquart, M. and Sörensen, S. (2003) 'Differences between caregivers and non-caregivers in psychological health and physical health: A meta-analysis', *Psychology and Aging*, 18:2, 250–267.

Plath, S. (1963) *The Bell Jar* (London: Faber and Faber, 2005).

Plumb, J. H. (1964) *Crisis in the Humanities* (London: Penguin Books).

Pogoriloffsky, A. (2011) *The Music of the Temporalists* (North Charleston, SC: CreateSpace).

Polkinghorne, D. E. (1988) *Narrative Knowing and the Human Sciences* (Albany: SUNY Press).

Popper, K. (1982) 'Science: Conjectures and refutations', in P. Grim (ed.) *The Philosophy of Science and the Occult* (Albany: New York State University Press), pp. 87–93.

Priest, H., Roberts, P. and Woods, L. (2002) 'An overview of three different approaches to the interpretation of qualitative data. Part 1: Theoretical issues', *Nurse Researcher*, 10:1, 30–42.

Prince, G. (1991) *Dictionary of Narratology* (Aldershot: Scholar Press).

Proctor, S. (2004) 'Playing politics: Community Music Therapy and the therapeutic redistribution of music capital for mental health', in M. Pavlicevic and G. Ansdell (eds) *Community Music Therapy* (London: Jessica Kingsley), pp. 214–232.

Propp, V. (1968) *Morphology of the Folktale* (2nd ed., trans. by L. Scott. Austin: University of Texas Press).

Puig, A., Lee, S. M., Goodwin, L. and Sherrard, P. A. D. (2006) 'The efficacy of creative arts therapies to enhance emotional expression, spirituality, and psychological well-being of newly diagnosed Stage I and Stage II breast cancer patients: A preliminary study', *The Arts in Psychotherapy*, 33, 218–228.

Ramachandran, V. S. and Hirstein, W. (1999) 'The science of art: A neurological theory of aesthetic experience', *Journal of Consciousness Studies*, 6:6–7, 15–51.

Ramazanoglu, C. (1992) 'On feminist methodology: Male reason versus female empowerment', *Sociology*, 26, 207–212.

Ray, R. (1998) *A Certain Age* (London: Penguin).

Read, J. and Reynolds, J. (eds) (1996) *Speaking Our Minds: An Anthology of Personal Experiences of Mental Distress and Its Consequences* (Basingstoke: Macmillan Press).

Reavey, P. (ed.) (2011) *Visual Methods in Psychology* (Hove: Psychology Press).

Reeves, S., Macmillan, K. and Van Soeren, M. (2010) 'Leadership of interprofessional health and social care teams: A socio-historical analysis', *Journal of Nursing Management*, 18, 258–264.

Repper, J. and Perkins, R. (2003) *Social Inclusion and Recovery* (Oxford: Baillière Tindall).

Reynolds, F. (2010) 'Colour and communion: Exploring the influences of visual art-making as a leisure activity on older women's subjective well-being', *Journal of Ageing Studies*, 24, 135–143.

Rich, J. A. and Grey, C. M. (2003) 'Qualitative research on trauma surgery: Getting beyond the numbers', *World Journal of Surgery*, 27, 957–961.

Richardson, B. (1997) *Unlikely Stories: Causality and the Nature of Modern Narrative* (Newark, DE: University of Delaware Press).

Rieger, B. (ed.) (1994) *Dionysus in Literature: Essays on Literary Madness* (Bowling Green, OH: Bowling Green State University Popular Press).

Riessman, C. K. (1993) *Narrative Analysis* (Thousand Oaks, CA: Sage).

—— (2002) 'Analysis of personal narratives', in J. F. Gubrium and J. A. Holstein (eds) *Handbook of Interview Research: Context and Method* (Thousand Oaks, CA: Sage), pp. 695–710.

Rietveld, T., Van Hout, R. and Ernestus, M. (2004) 'Pitfalls in corpus research', *Computers and the Humanities*, 38, 343–362.

Rimmon-Kenan, S. (2002) *Narrative Fiction* (2nd ed. London: Routledge).

Robbins, C. (2005) *A Journey into Creative Music Therapy* (University Park, IL: Barcelona Publishers).

Roberts, S., Camic, P. M. and Springham, N. (2011) 'New roles for art galleries: Art-viewing as a community intervention for family carers of people with mental health problems', *Arts and Health: An International Journal for Research, Policy and Practice*, 3:2, 146–159.

Rogers, A. and Pilgrim, D. (2003) *Mental Health and Inequality* (Basingstoke: Palgrave Macmillan).

Rolfe, A., Mienczakowski, J. and Morgan, S. (1995) 'A dramatic experience in mental health nursing education', *Nurse Education Today*, 15:3, 224–227.

Ross, C. (2012) *Words for Wellbeing* (Cumbria: Cumbria Partnership NHS Trust).

Ross, C. A., Schroder, E. and Ness, L. (2013) 'Dissociation and symptoms of culture-bound syndromes in North America: A preliminary study', *Journal of Trauma and Dissociation*, 14, 224–235.

Ross, M. (1994) 'Maggy Ross', in L. Pembroke (ed.) *Self-Harm: Perspectives from Personal Experience* (London: Survivors Speak Out).

Rossiter, K., Kontos, P., Colantonio, A., Gilbert, J., Gray, J. and Keightley, M. (2008) 'Staging data: Theatre as a tool for analysis and knowledge transfer in health research', *Social Science and Medicine*, 66:1, 130–146.

Rothschild, B. and Rand, M. (2006) *Help for the Helper: The Psychophysiology of Compassion Fatigue and Vicarious Trauma* (New York: W. W. Norton).

Rubin, J. (2005) *Artful Therapy* (Hoboken, NJ: John Wiley and Sons).

Rudow, B. (1999) 'Stress and burnout in the teaching profession: European studies, issues, and research perspectives', in R. Vandenberghe and A. M. Huberman (eds) *Understanding and Preventing Teacher Burnout: A Sourcebook of International Research and Practice* (Cambridge, UK: Cambridge University Press), pp. 38–58.

Rutledge, M. (2004) *Dance as Research: The Experience of Surrender* (Unpublished doctoral dissertation, University of Alberta).

Ruud, E. (1998) *Music Therapy: Improvisation, Communication and Culture* (University Park, IL: Barcelona Publishers).

Sackett, D. L., Rosenberg, W. M. C., Muir Grey, J. A., Haynes, R. B. and Richardson, W. S. (1996) 'Evidence-based medicine: What it is and what it isn't', *British Medical Journal*, 312, 71–72.

Sacks, O. (1985) *The Man Who Mistook his Wife for a Hat* (London: Picador, 2007).

Salter, K., Hellings, C., Foley, N. and Teasell, R. (2008) 'The experience of living with stroke: A qualitative meta-synthesis', *Journal of Rehabilitative Medicine*, 40, 595–602.

Sánchez Camus, R. (2009) 'The problem of application: Aesthetics in creativity and health', *Health Care Analysis*, 17:4, 345–355.

Sandel, S. L., Judge, J. O., Landry, N., Faria, L., Ouellette, R. and Majczak, M. (2005) 'Dance and movement program improves quality-of-life measures in breast cancer survivors', *Cancer Nursing*, 28:4, 301–309.

Sandelowski, M. (1991) 'Telling stories: Narrative approaches in qualitative research', *Journal of Nursing Scholarship*, 23:3, 161–166.

Sandelowski, M., Docherty, S. and Emden, C. (1997) 'Focus on qualitative methods. Qualitative metasynthesis: Issues and techniques', *Research in Nursing and Health*, 20, 365–371.

Sarbin, T. (1986) *Narrative Psychology: The Storied Nature of Human Conduct* (New York: Praeger).

—— (1997) 'The poetics of identity', *Theory and Psychology*, 7:1, 67–82.

Sass, L. (1992) *Madness and Modernism: Insanity in the Light of Modern Art, Literature and Thought* (Cambridge, MA: Harvard University Press).

Savin-Baden, M. and Fisher, A. (2002) 'Negotiating "honesties" in the research process', *British Journal of Occupational Therapy*, 65:4, 191–193.

Scarry, E. (1985) *The Body in Pain: The Making and Unmaking of the World* (Oxford: Oxford University Press).

Schaff, P. B., Isken, S. and Tager, R. M. (2011) 'From contemporary art to core clinical skills: Observation, interpretation, and meaning-making in a complex environment', *Academic Medicine*, 86:10, 1272–1276.

Schmid, T. (2004) 'Meanings of creativity within occupational therapy practice', *Australian Occupational Therapy Journal*, 51, 80–88.

Schutz, A. (1962) *The Problem of Social Reality: Collected Papers I* (The Hague: Martinus Nijhoff).

Schwartz, H. (1989) 'The three body problem and the end of the world', in M. Feher, R. Nadaff and N. Tazi (eds) *Fragments for a History of the Human Body: Part 2* (New York: Zone Books), pp. 411–420.

Schwarz, M. R. and Wojtczak, A. (2002) 'Global minimum essential requirements: A road towards competence-oriented medical education', *Medical Teacher*, 24, 125–129.

Seale, C. (2006) 'Gender accommodation in online cancer support groups', *Health*, 10, 345–360.

Seale, C., Boden, S., Williams, S., Lowe, P. and Steinberg, D. (2007) 'Media constructions of sleep and sleep disorders: A study of UK national newspapers', *Social Science and Medicine*, 65, 418–430.

Secker, J., Hacking, S., Spandler, H., Kent, L. and Shenton, J. (2007) *Mental Health, Social Inclusion and Arts: Developing the Evidence Base. Final Report* (Department of Health, UClan and Anglia Ruskin University).

Seligman, A. B. (2010) 'Ritual and sincerity: Certitude and the other', *Philosophy and Social Criticism*, 36:1, 9–39.

Sered, S. (1999) '"You are a number, not a human being": Israeli breast cancer patients' experiences with medical establishment', *Medical Anthropology Quarterly*, 13:2, 223–252.

Shan, H. H. (2000) 'Culture bound psychiatric disorders associated with qigong practice in China', *Hong Kong Journal of Psychiatry*, 10:3, 10–14.

Shankar, P. R. (2008) 'A need to develop medical humanities in Nepal', *Kathmandu University Medical Journal*, 6:1, 146–147.

Shaw, A. B. (2002) 'Depressive illness delayed Hamlet's revenge', *Medical Humanities*, 28, 92–96.

Shepherd, G., Boardman, J. and Slade, M. (2008) *Making Recovery a Reality* (London: (Sainsbury Centre for Mental Health).

Showalter, E. (1987) *The Female Malady: Women, Madness and English Culture 1830–1980* (London: Virago).

Sinding, C. (2014) 'Metaphors in a patient's narrative: Picturing good care', *Ethics and Social Welfare*, 8:1, 57–74.

Skyman, E., Sjostrom, H. T. and Hellstrom, E. (2010) 'Patients' experiences of being infected with MRSA at a hospital and subsequently source isolated', *Scandinavian Journal of Caring Sciences*, 24:1, 101–107.

Slade, D., Thomas-Connor, I. and Tsao, T. M. (2008) 'When nursing meets English: Using a pathography to develop nursing student's culturally competent selves', *Nursing Education Perspectives*, 29:3, 151–155.

Small, C. (1998) *Musicking: The Meanings of Performing and Listening* (Middletown, CT: Wesleyan University Press).

Smeijsters, H. and Gorry, C. (2006) 'The treatment of aggression using arts therapies in forensic psychiatry: Results of a qualitative inquiry', *The Arts in Psychotherapy*, 33, 37–58.

Smith, B. H. (1981) 'Narrative versions, narrative theories', in W. J. T. Mitchell (ed.) *On Narrative* (Chicago, IL: University of Chicago Press), pp. 209–232.

Smith, J. E. (1969) 'Time, times, and the "right time": *Chronos* and *kairos*', *The Monist*, 53, 1–13.

Snowden, R., Thompson, P. and Troscianko, T. (2006) *Basic Vision: An Introduction to Visual Perception* (Oxford: Oxford University Press).

Sommer, C. A., Kholomeydek, N., Meacham, P., Thomas, Z., Bryant, M. L. and Derrick, E. C. (2012) 'The supervisee with a thousand faces: Using stories to enhance supervision', *Journal of Poetry Therapy*, 25:3, 151–163.

Soundy, A., Smith, B., Cressy, F. and Webb, L. (2010) 'The experience of spinal cord injury: Using Frank's narrative types to enhance physiotherapy undergraduates' understanding', *Physiotherapy*, 96, 52–58.

Spandler, H., Secker, J., Kent, L., Hacking, S. and Shenton, J. (2007) 'Catching life: The contribution of arts initiatives to "recovery" approaches in mental health', *Journal of Psychiatric and Mental Health Nursing*, 14:8, 791–799.

Speedy, J. (2000) 'Consulting with gargoyles: Applying narrative ideas and practices in counselling supervision', *European Journal of Psychotherapy, Counselling, and Health*, 3, 419–431.

Stanley, L. and Wise, S. (1983) *Breaking Out: Feminist Consciousness and Feminist Research* (London: Routledge).

Staricoff, R. (2004) *A Study of the Effects of Visual and Performing Arts in Healthcare for Chelsea and Westminster Hospital*. www.publicartonline.org.uk/resources/research/documents/ChelseaAndWestminsterResearchproject.pdf, accessed 30 March 2014.

Stempsey, W. E. (1999) 'The quarantine of philosophy in medical education: Why teaching the humanities may not produce humane physicians', *Medicine, Health Care and Philosophy*, 2, 3–9.

Stetler, R. (2010) 'Experience-based, body-anchored qualitative research interviewing', *Qualitative Health Research*, 20:6, 859–867.

Stickley, T. and Duncan, K. (2010) 'Learning about community arts', in V. Tischler (ed.) *Mental Health Psychiatry and the Arts* (London: Radcliffe Publishing), pp. 101–110.

Stige, B. (2002) *Culture-Centered Music Therapy* (University Park, IL: Barcelona Publishers).

—— (2012) 'Health musicking: A perspective on music and health as action and performance', in R. MacDonald, G. Kreutz and L. Mitchell (eds) *Music, Health, and Wellbeing* (Oxford: Oxford University Press), pp. 183–195.

Stoudt, B. G., Fox, M. and Fine, M. (2012) 'Contesting privilege with critical participatory action research', *Journal of Social Issues*, 68:1, 178–193.

Street, G., James, R. and Cutt, H. (2007) 'The relationship between organised physical recreation and mental health', *Health Promotion Journal of Australia*, 18, 236–239.

Stronach, I. and MacLure, M. (1997) *Educational Research Undone: The Postmodern Embrace* (Buckingham: Open University Press).

Styron, W. (1990) *Darkness Visible: A Memoir of Madness* (London: Vintage Books, 2004).

Suryani, L. K. and Jensen, G. D. (1993) *Trance and Possession in Bali* (Oxford: Oxford University Press).

Suzuki, L. and Calzo, J. (2004) 'The search for peer advice in cyberspace: An examination of online teen bulletin boards about health and sexuality', *Applied Developmental Psychology*, 25, 685–698.

Swanson, G. E. (1992) 'Doing things together: Some basic forms of agency and structure in collective action and some explanations', *Social Psychology Quarterly*, 55:2, 94–117.

Swartz, L. (2011) 'Dissociation and spirit possession in non-Western countries', in V. Sinason (ed.) *Attachment, Trauma and Multiplicity: Working with Dissociative Identity Disorder* (London: Routledge), pp. 63–71.

Tarzi, P., Kennedy, P., Stone, S. and Evans, M . (2001) 'Methicillin-resistant *Staphylococcus aureus*: Psychological impact of hospitalization and isolation in an older adult population', *Journal of Hospital Infection*, 49, 250–254.

Tatar, M. (1999) *The Classic Fairy Tales* (New York: W. W. Norton).

Taussig, M. (1977) 'The genesis of capitalism amongst a South American peasantry: Devil's labour and the baptism of money', *Comparative Studies in Society and History*, 19:2, 130–155.

Tegner, I., Fox, J., Philipp, R. and Thorne, P. (2009) 'Evaluating the use of poetry to improve well-being and emotional resilience in cancer patients', *Journal of Poetry Therapy*, 22:3, 121–131.

Tew, J. (2012) 'Recovery capital: What enables a sustainable recovery from mental health difficulties?' *European Journal of Social Work*, DOI: 10.1080/13691457.2012.687713.

The National Alliance for Caregiving and AARP (2009) *Caregiving in the U. S.* (Washington, DC: National Alliance for Caregiving).

The Reading Agency (2012) 'Mood Boosting Books for Carers', http://readingagency.org.uk/adults/tips/your-mood-boosting-recommendations-for-carers.html, accessed 3 April 2014.

The Telegraph (2009) 'Reading "can help reduce stress"', *The Telegraph*, 30 March 2009, www.telegraph.co.uk/health/healthnews/5070874/Reading-can-help-reduce stress.html, accessed 1 December 2010.

Thompson, M. and Blair, S. E. E. (1998) 'Creative arts in occupational therapy: Ancient history or contemporary practise?' *Occupational Therapy International*, 5:1, 48–64.

Tischler, V. (in press) *Silenced:* the impact of mental health themed artwork in a workplace setting. *Journal of Applied Arts and Health*.

Tischler, V. (ed.) (2010) *Mental Health, Psychiatry and The Arts: A Teaching Handbook* (Oxon: Radcliffe Publishing).

Tischler, V., Pratten, M. and Ben-Zenou, H. (2010) 'Seeing within: Art and the study of anatomy', in G. Baker (ed.) *Teaching for Integrative Learning: Innovations in University Practice, Vol. 4* (Nottingham: Centre for Integrative Learning), pp. 143–151. www.heacademy.ac.uk/assets/documents/employability/CIL_Case_Studies_volume_4.pdf, accessed 30 March 2014.

Tischler, V., Chopra, A., Nixon, N. and McCormack, L. (2011) 'Loss and tomorrow's doctors: How the humanities can contribute to personal and professional development', *International Journal of Person-Centered Medicine*, 1:3, 547–552.

Tjørnhøj-Thomsen, T. and Hansen, H. P. (2013) 'The ritualization of rehabilitation', *Medical Anthropology*, 32, 266–285.

Tortora, S. (2009) 'Dance/movement psychotherapy in early childhood treatment', in S. Chaiklin and H. Wengrower (eds) *The Art and Science of Dance/Movement Therapy: Life is Dance* (New York: Routledge), pp. 159–180.

Toulmin, S. (1978) 'The Mozart of psychology', *The New York Review of Books*, 28 September, 25:14, 51–57.

Trousseau, A. (1869) *Lectures on Clinical Medicine, Introduction, Vol. 2* (London: The New Sydenham Society).

Turner, V. (1969) *The Ritual Process* (Chicago, IL: Aldine).

—— (1974) *Drama, Fields and Metaphors: Symbolic Action in Human Society* (Ithaca, NY and London: Cornell University Press).

Upshur, R. E. G., Vandenkerkhof, E. G. and Goel, V. (2001) 'Meaning and measurement: An inclusive model of evidence in health care', *Journal of Evaluation in Clinical Practice*, 7, 91–96.

US Department of Health and Human Services (2008) 'The Registered Nurse Population: Findings from the 2004 national samples survey of registered nurses', http://bhpr.hrsa.gov/healthworkforce/rnsurvey04/, accessed 7 February 2009.

van Gennep, A. (1960) [1909] *The Rites of Passage* (Chicago, IL: Chicago University Press).

Vandell, D. L., Pierce, K. M. and Dadisman, K. (2005) 'Out-of-school settings as a developmental context for children and youth', *Advances in Child Development and Behavior*, 33, 43–77.

Vega, S. (1987) *Luka* [original song].

Venkataramaiah, V., Mallikarjunaiah, M., Chandra, C. R., Rao, C. K. and Reddy, G. N. (1981) 'Possession syndrome: An epidemiological study in West Karnataka', *Indian Journal of Psychiatry*, 23, 213–218.

Venkatasalu, M. E., Seymour, J. E. and Arthur, A. (2014) 'Dying at home: A qualitative study of the perspectives of older South Asians living in the United Kingdom', *Palliative Medicine*, 28:3, 264–272.

Visholm, T. (2010) *It's Impossible to Worry and Be Creative at the Same Time* (Unpublished BMedSci dissertation, University of Nottingham).

Vygotsky, L. S. (1978) *Mind in Society: The Development of the Higher Psychological Processes* (Cambridge, MA: Harvard University Press).

Wallace, A. (1966) *Religion: An Anthropological View* (New York: Random House).

Wallace, S. (2008) 'Governing humanity', *Journal of Medical Humanities*, 29:1, 27–32.

Warner, D. and Spandler, H. (2012) 'New strategies for practice-based evidence: A focus on self-harm', *Qualitative Research in Psychology*, 9, 13–26.

Wartofsky, M. (1983) 'The child's construction of the world and the world's construction of the child: From historical epistemology to historical psychology', in F. S. Kessel and A. W. Sigel (eds) *The Child and Other Cultural Inventions* (New York: Praeger), pp. 188–215.

Weber, A. M. and Haen, C. (2005) *Clinical Applications of Drama Therapy in Child and Adolescent Treatment* (London: Routledge).

White, M. and Robson, M. (2011) 'Finding sustainability: University–community collaborations focused on arts in health', *Gateways: International Journal of Community Research and Engagement*, 4, 48–64.

Whitehead, A. (2014) 'The medical humanities: A literary perspective', in V. Bates, A. Bleakley and S. Goodman (eds) *Medicine, Health and The Arts: Approaches to Medical Humanities* (Oxon: Routledge), pp. 107–127.

Whooley, O. (2010) 'Diagnostic ambivalence: Psychiatric workarounds and the Diagnostic and Statistical Manual of Mental Disorders', *Sociology of Health and Illness*, 32:3, 452–469.

Widder, J. (2004) 'The origins of medical evidence: Communication and experimentation', *Medicine, Health Care and Philosophy*, 7, 99–104.

Wijesinghe, C. P., Dissanayake, S. A. W. and Mendis, N. (1976) 'Possession trance in a semi-urban community in Sri Lanka', *Australian and New Zealand Journal of Psychiatry*, 11, 93–100.

Wilcox, D. (1994) *Chet Baker's Unsung Swan Song* [original song], in D. Wilcox (1999) *The David Wilcox Song Book* (Milwaukee, WI: Hal Leonard).

Williams, C. (2001) 'Use of written cognitive-behavioural therapy self-help materials to treat depression', *Advances in Psychiatric Treatment*, 7, 233–240.

Willow Breast Cancer Support Canada (2010) *Managing Your Cancer Care: A Self Advocacy Guide for Breast Cancer Patients* (Toronto, ON: Willow Breast Cancer Support Canada).

Wittchen, H. U., Jacobi, F., Rehm, J., Gustavsson, A., Svensson, M., Jönsson, B., et al. (2011) 'The size and burden of mental disorders and other disorders of the brain in Europe 2010', *European Neuropsychopharmacology*, 21:9, 655–679.

Wittgenstein, L. (1953) *Philosophical Investigations* (trans. by G. E. M. Anscombe. Oxford: Blackwell).

Wood, M., Ferlie, E. and Fitzgerald, L. (1998) 'Achieving clinical behaviour change: A case of becoming indeterminate', *Social Science and Medicine*, 47, 1729–1738.

Woods, A. (2011) *The Sublime Object of Psychiatry: Schizophrenia in Clinical and Cultural Theory* (Oxford: Oxford University Press).

Woolliscroft, J. O. and Phillips, R. (2003) 'Medicine as a performing art: A worthy metaphor', *Medical Education*, 37, 934–939.

World Health Organization (WHO) (2005) *Mental Health: Facing the Challenges, Building Solutions* (Copenhagen: World Health Organization, Europe).

Wurtzel, E. (1994) *Prozac Nation: Young and Depressed in America – A Memoir* (London: Quartet Books).

Yalom, I. (1989) *Love's Executioner and Other Tales of Psychotherapy* (London: Penguin).

Zeki, S. (2000) *Inner Vision* (Oxford: Oxford University Press).

Zipes, J. (2006) *Why Fairy Tales Stick: The Evolution and Relevance of a Genre* (New York: Routledge).

Zuckerkandl, V. (1956) *Sound and Symbol* (New York: Bollingen).

Index

190 *Index*

Made in the USA
San Bernardino, CA
27 August 2017